C'est quoi sur l'ardoise?

What's on the menu tonight?

Easy recipes from a small
restaurant in France...

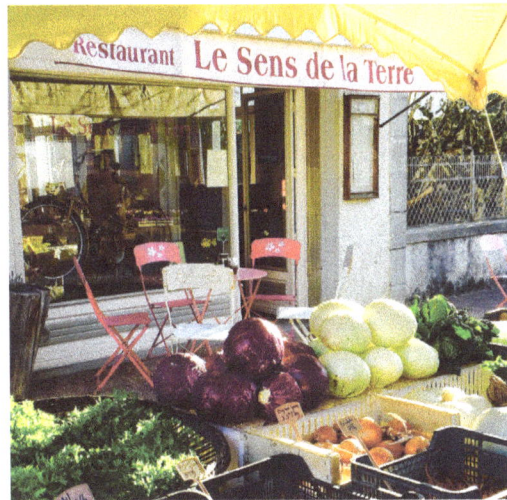

MOSAÏQUEPRESS

Published in 2020

MOSAÏQUE PRESS

Registered office:
70 Priory Road
Kenilworth
Warwickshire, UK
CV8 1LQ

Also available in French
(ISBN 978-1-906852-56-6)

ISBN 978-1-906852-57-3

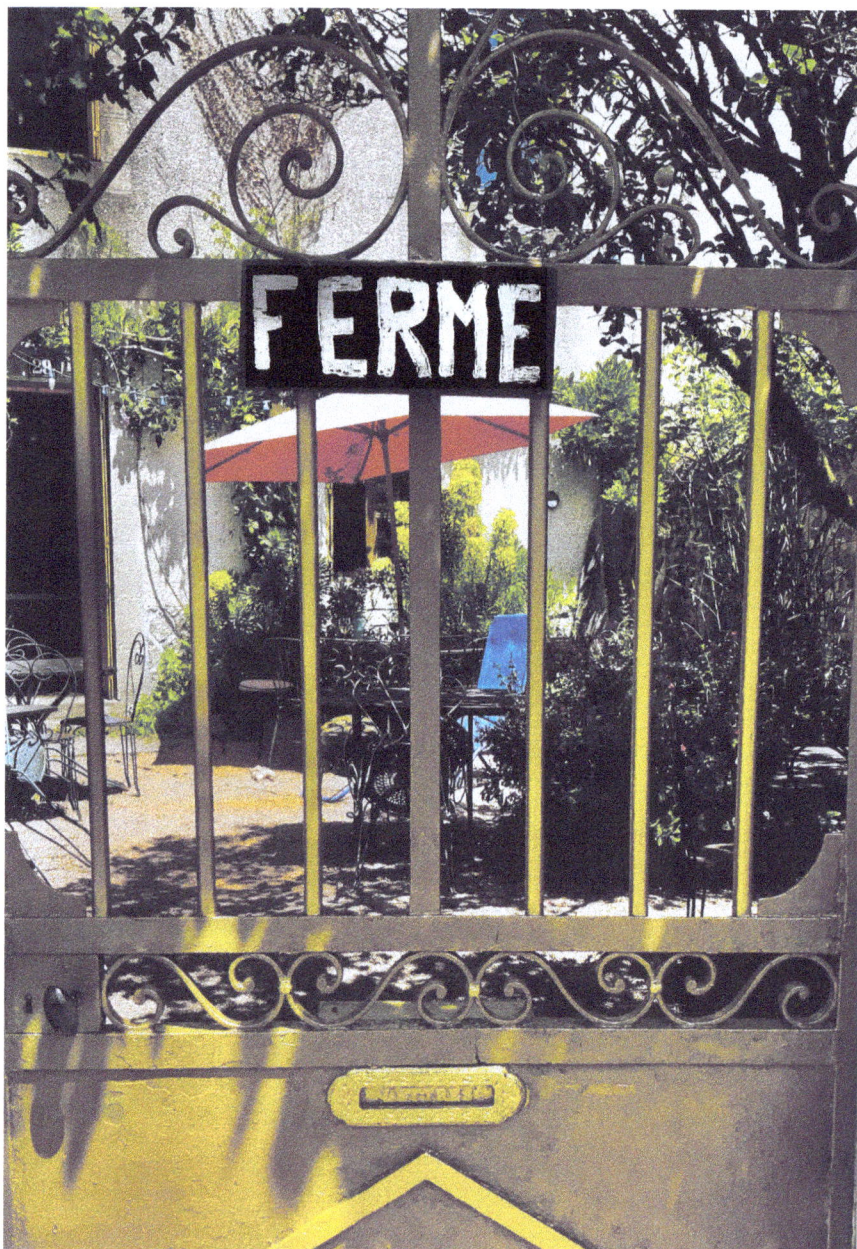

16 March 2020
11.23am
Le Sens de la Terre Restaurant
24360 Piégut-Pluviers

"What's on the menu today, Claire?"

"I don't know Leo, I've had other things on my mind since yesterday."

"Me too, but I'm hungry anyway."

The phone rings. "Le Sens de la Terre, Claire – hello."

"Is it true that you and all other restaurants are closed as of last night?"

"Yes, it was a big surprise and a shock for us too!"

"So my reservation for today is cancelled?"

"Yes, we're so sorry!"

"But what will I eat today?"

"Well, if you have a few ingredients in your kitchen – potatoes, eggs, vegetables – you can make a tasty meal..."

"Okay, thank you, I'll try to cook for myself."

"Have fun and enjoy your meal! Have a good day."

That's how it all started... That's what inspired us to post recipes on Facebook every day during the lockdown.

And now you have these recipes in your hands.

Bon appetit!

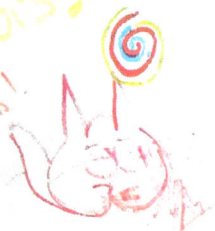
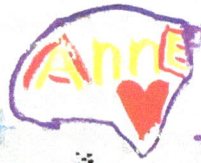
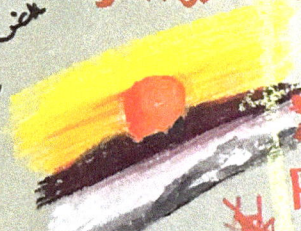
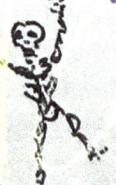

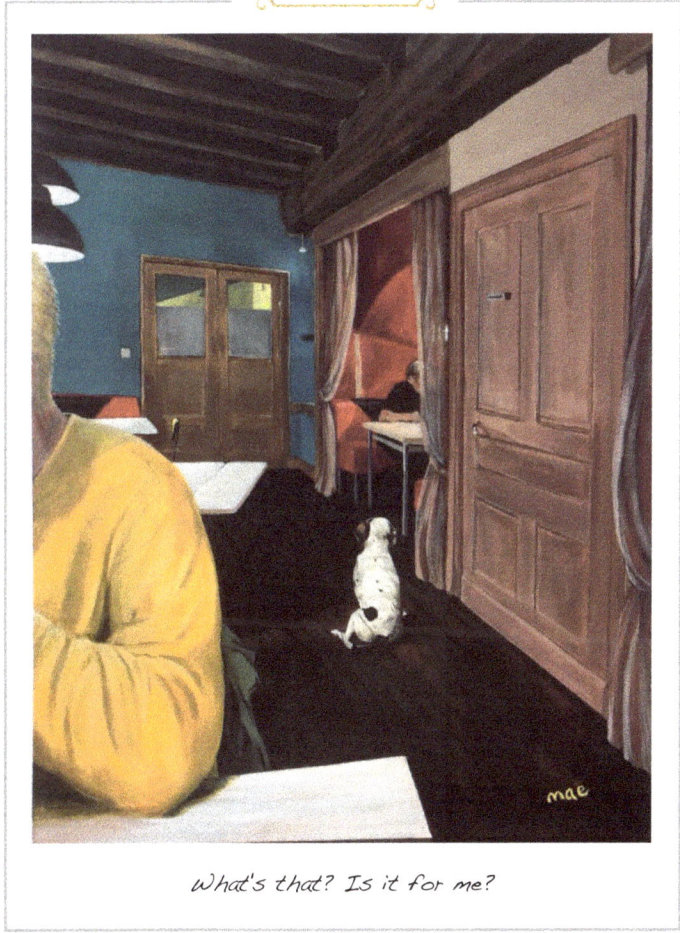

What's that? Is it for me?

A note on measures

tsp = teaspoon = approx 5ml
tbsp = tablespoon = approx 15ml
g = gram (250g = approx 1/2 lb)
kg = kilogram (1kg = 2.2 lb)
ml = mililitre (30ml = 1 fl oz)

For recipes with pastry, 250g
of flour is approx 2 cups

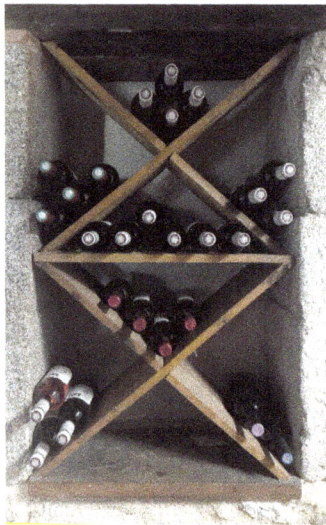

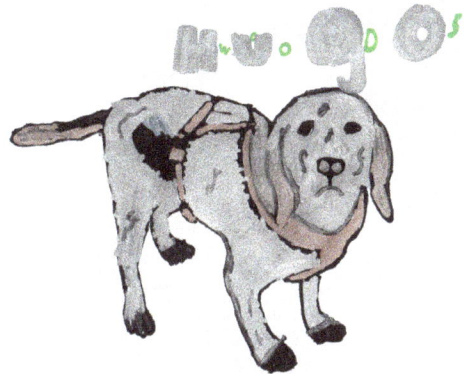

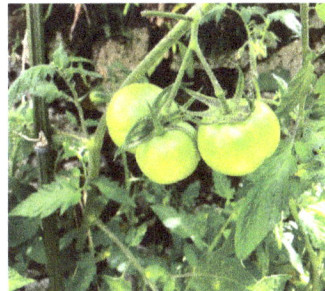

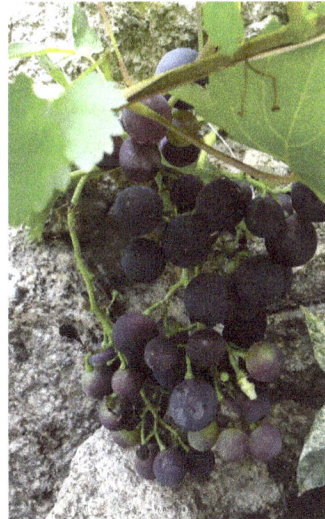

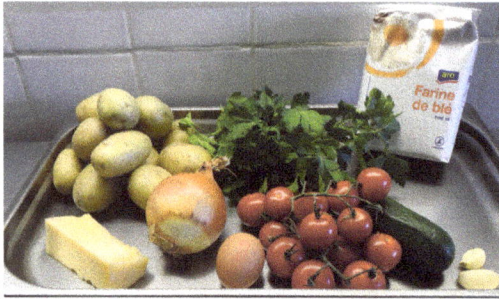

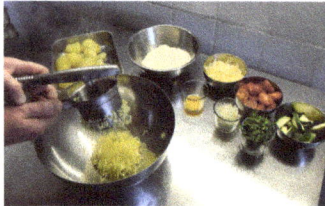

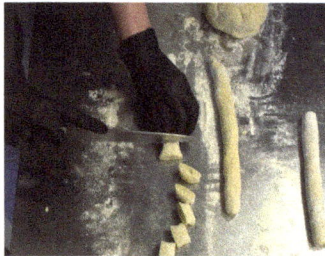

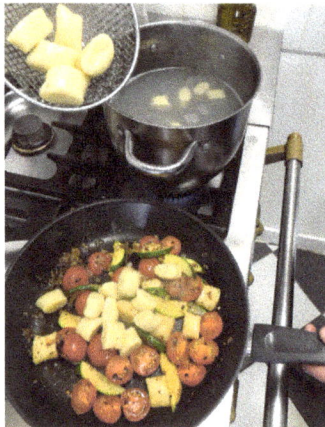

Spring gnocchis
(Serves 4)

1kg potatoes
250g flour
1 egg yolk, olive oil
Ground pepper, salt
Nutmeg
1 courgette
1 onion
1 clove of garlic (or more)
12 cherry tomatoes
Parsley
100g Parmesan cheese

Boil potatoes until soft, peel them and mash until smooth.

When the mash is cool, mix with the egg yolk and flour. Season to taste with salt, pepper and nutmeg. Roll into sausage shapes and cut into pieces of 1–2cm.

Next chop the onions, garlic, courgette and the cherry tomatoes, finely chop the parley and finely grate the Parmesan cheese.

Bring a pot of salted water to the boil and place the gnocchis in it to cook. When they rise to the surface, remove them from the water.

Lightly brown the onions, garlic and courgettes in a frying pan with some olive oil. Add the gnocchis and season with salt and pepper.

Serve with the chopped parsley and Parmesan.

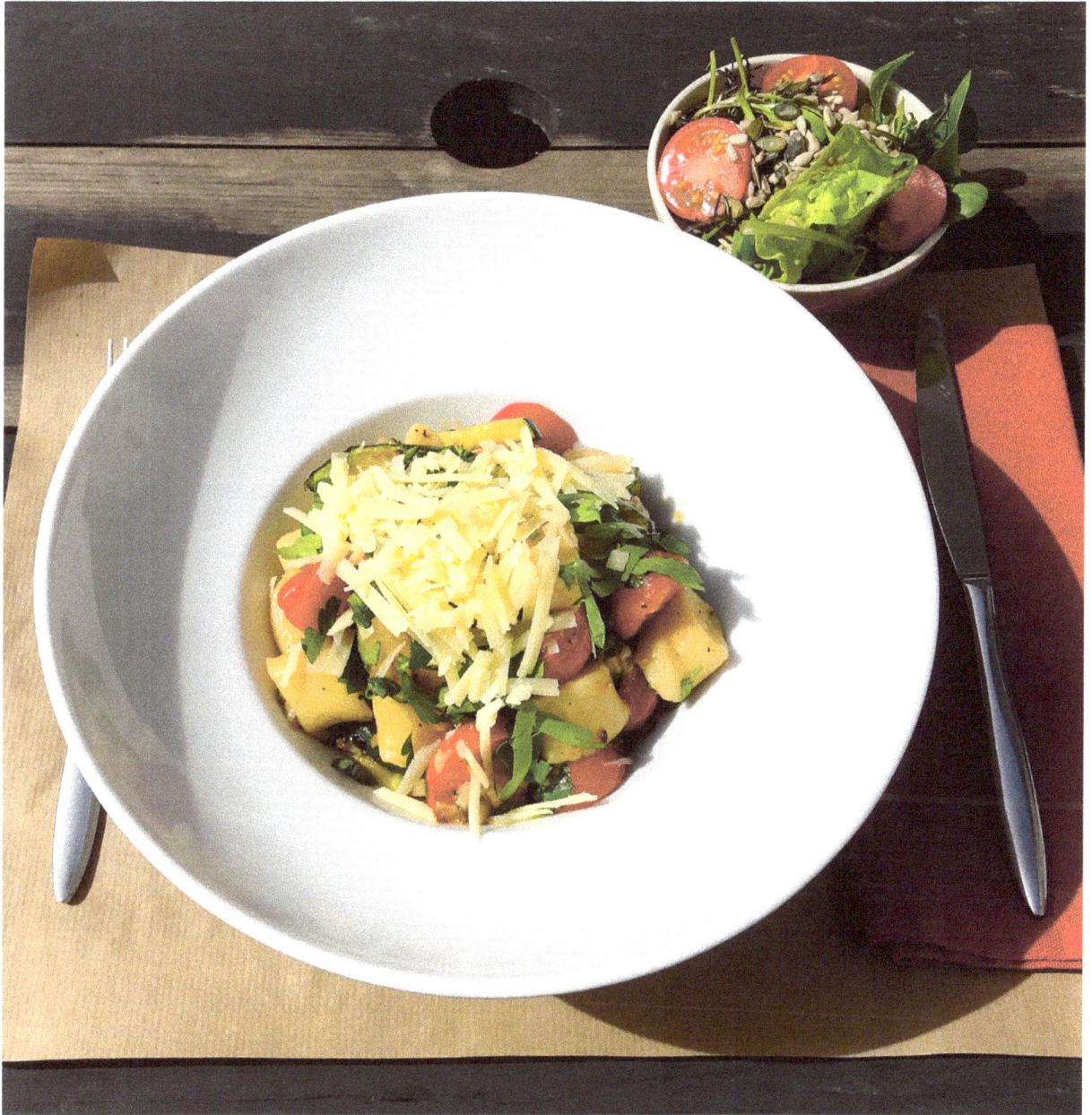

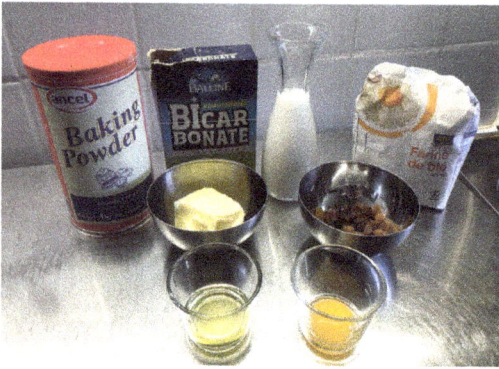

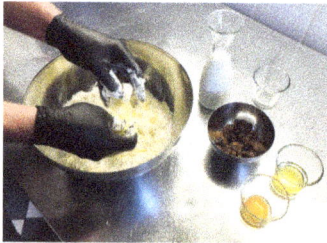

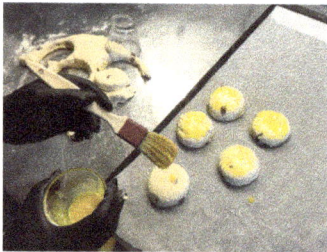

Scones
(makes 12)

500g flour
50g butter
6 tsp baking powder
1/2 tsp baking soda
1 egg, separated
50–75g raisins (optional)
220ml milk

Preheat your oven to 200°C.

Mix the flour, baking powder, baking soda and melted butter with your fingers in a bowl.

Add the raisins and egg white and knead in the milk little by little to form a smooth dough.

Roll out the dough to 1 1/2cm and cut out round pieces of approx 7cm with a sturdy cup or glass, floured.

Place the scones on a baking tray, brush with the egg yolk and bake for 15 min or until golden brown.

Serve with butter and strawberry preserve.

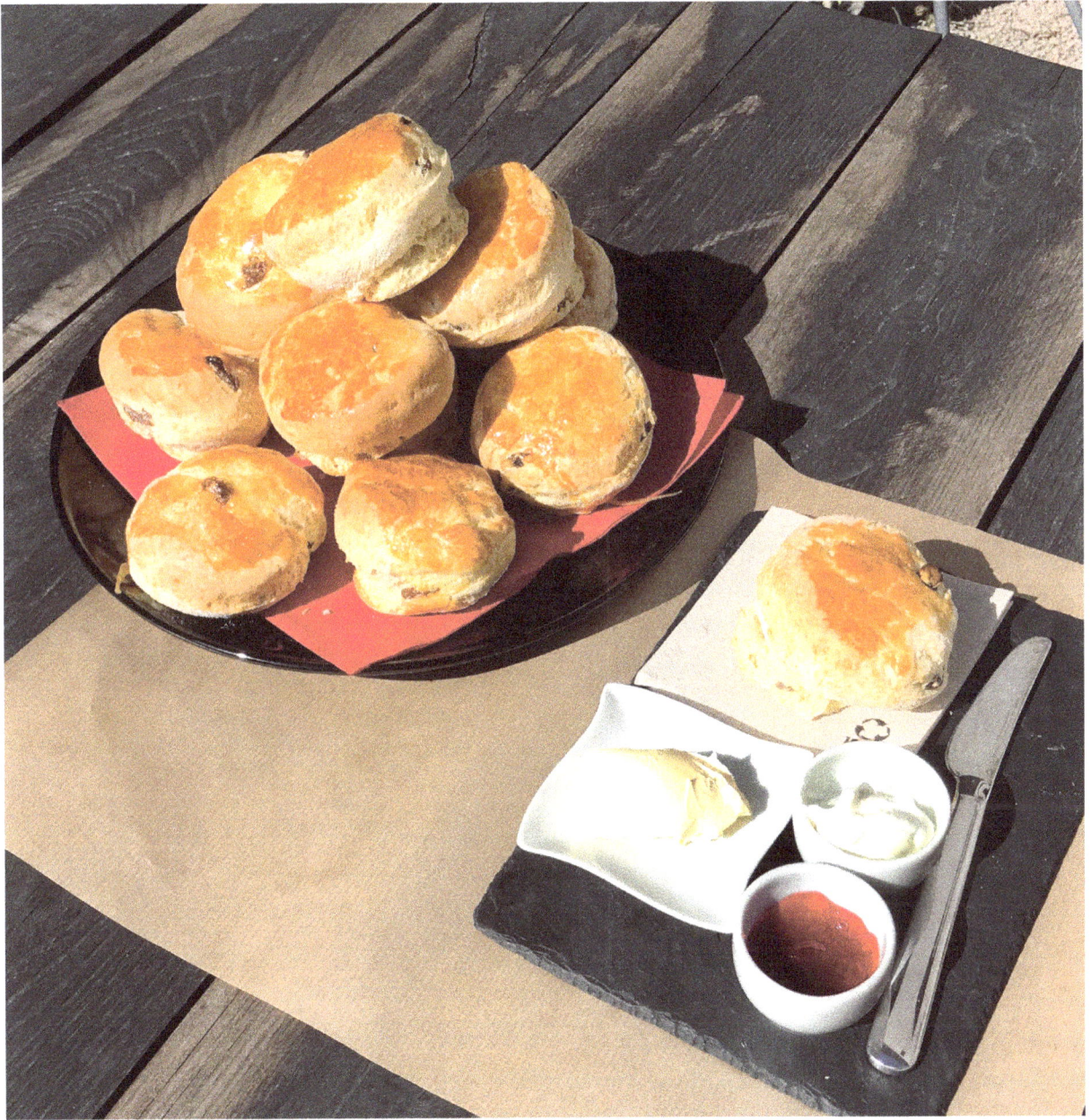

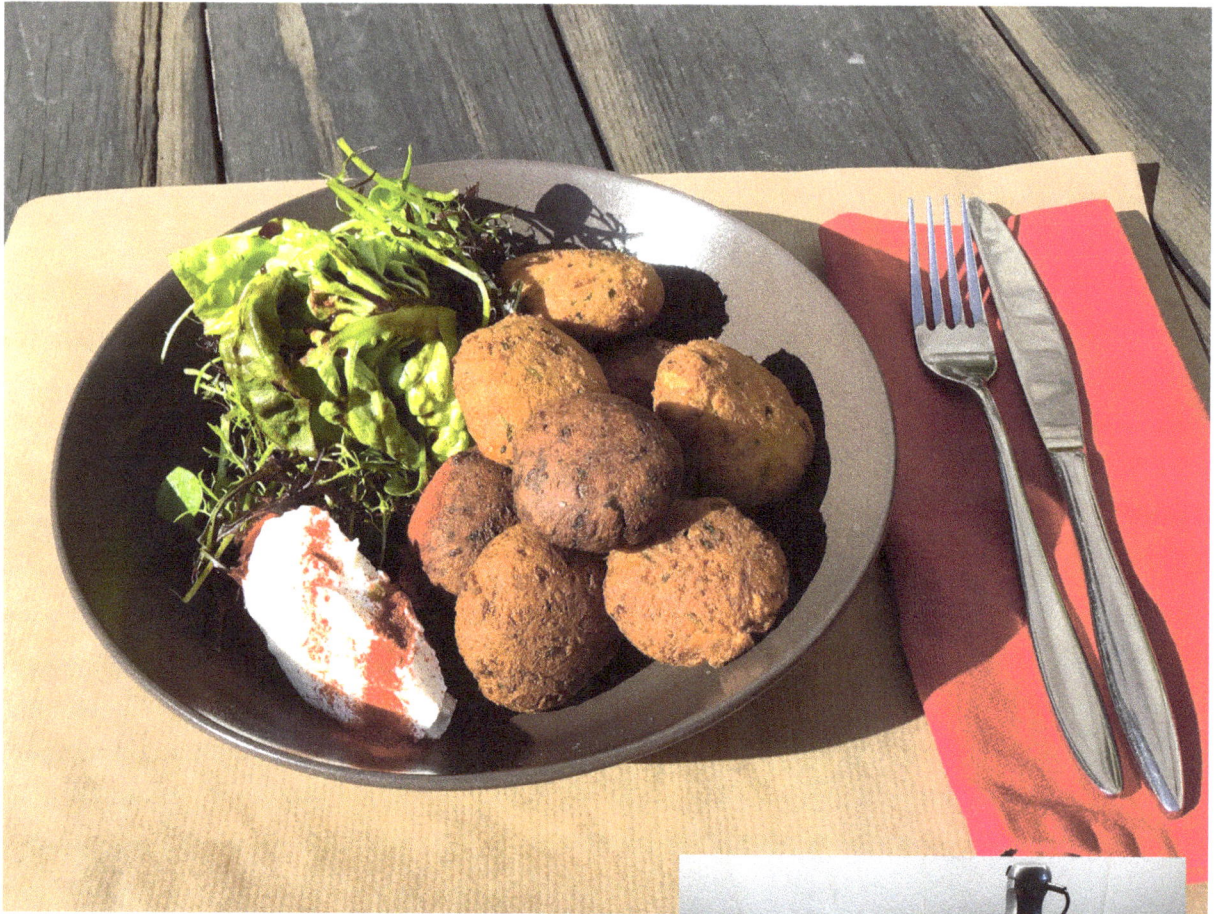

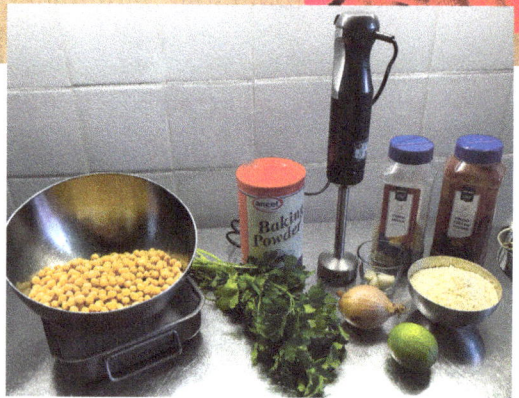

Falafels
(makes 15)

400g tinned chick peas, drained
and rinsed with cold water
150g chick pea flour
1 1/2 tsp baking powder
1 onion
2 garlic cloves
Parsley/coriander
Chilli powder
Salt and pepper
Cumin
Lime juice

Mix chick peas, herbs, garlic and onion with a purée
mixer to a smooth paste.

Add the chick pea flour, baking powder and season
with salt, pepper, cumin, lime juice and chilli powder
to your taste. If the mixture is too thin, add more chick
pea flour to obtain a firm consistency.

Leave to rest in the fridge for 30 min.

Pat the mixture into 15 even round slightly flat pieces.

Fry the falafels in hot oil (180°C) until golden brown.

Serve with tzatziki *(see recipe on Day 4)*
and a green salad.

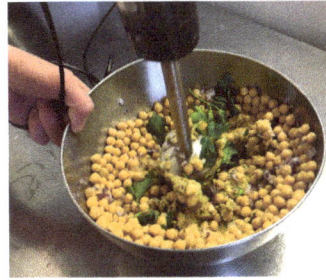

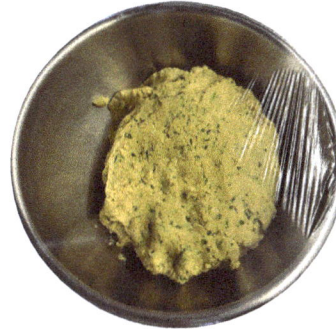

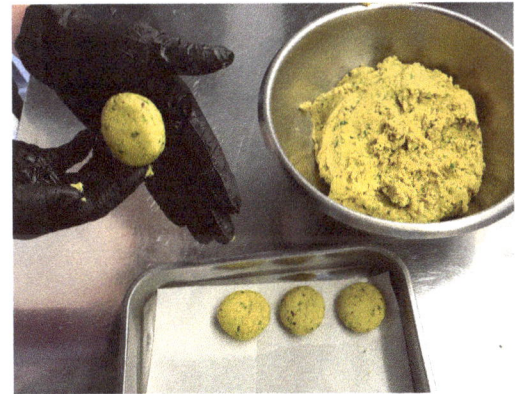

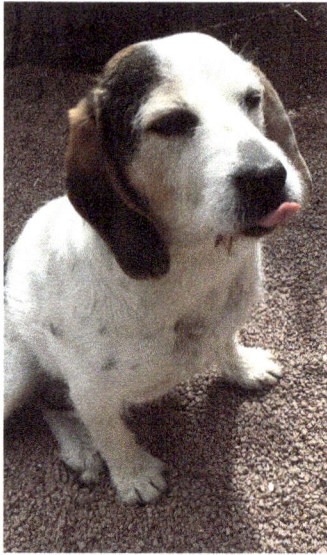

Tzatziki

300g Greek yoghurt
1/3 cucumber
1/2 onion, finely chopped
2 garlic cloves, finely chopped
20ml olive oil
Lime juice
Salt
Pepper
Cumin

Grate the cucumber, add a little salt and
leave until the water starts to separate
from the cucumber.

Press the water out in a kitchen towel and
place the cucumber back into a bowl
with the yogurt, onion and garlic.

Add olive oil and season with salt, pepper,
cumin and lime juice to taste.

Perfect with falafels
or just plain pita bread.

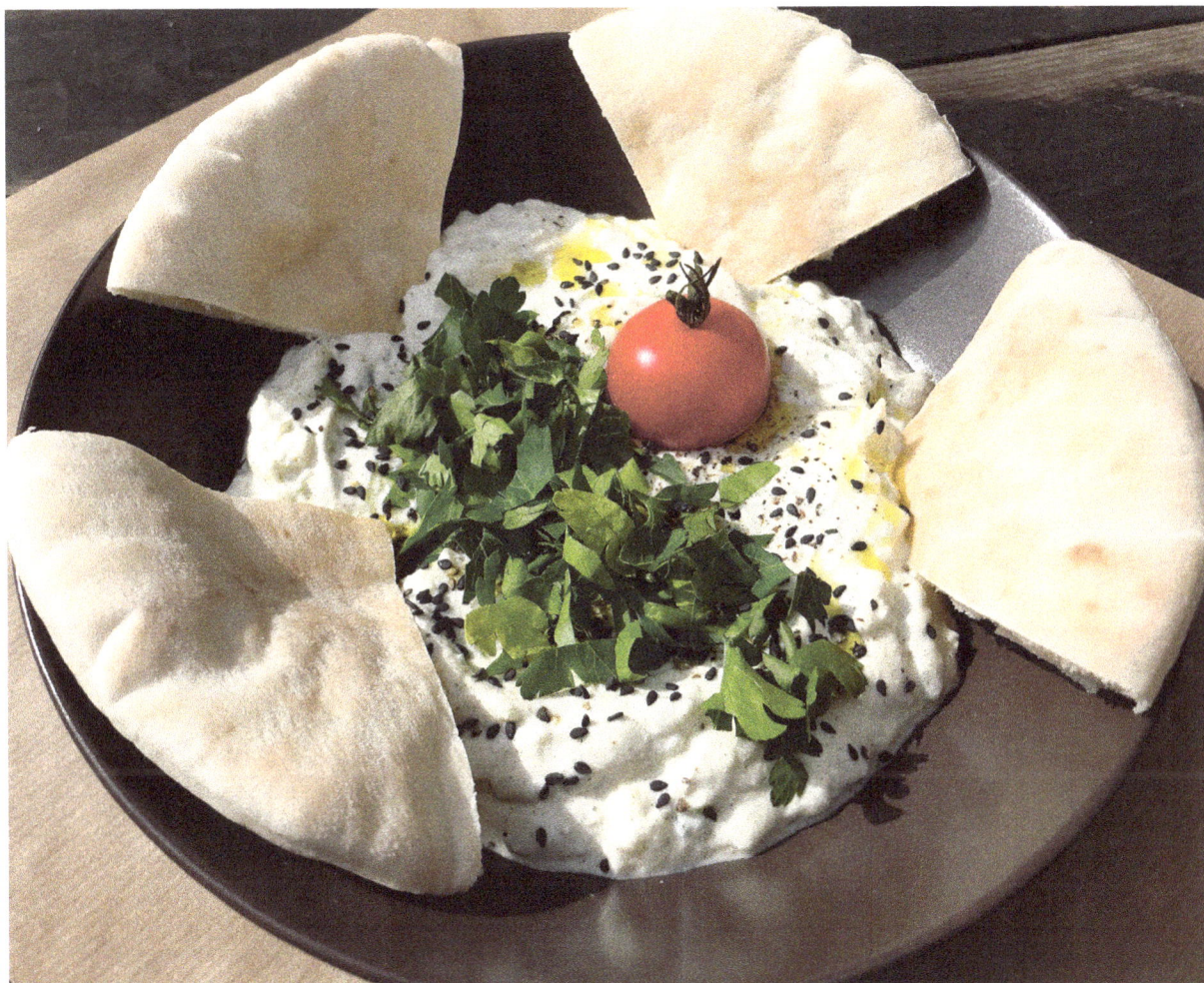

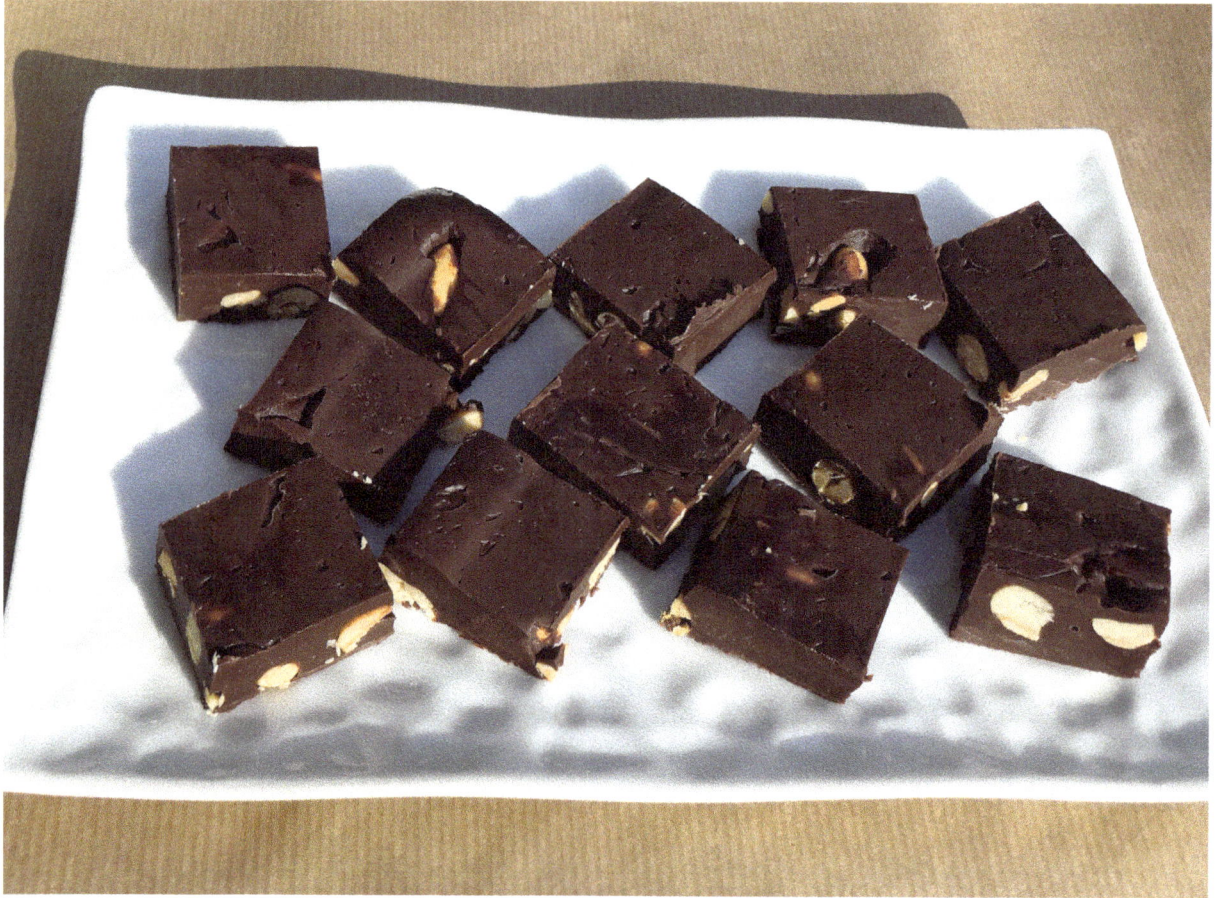

Chocolate-peanut fudge

300g dark chocolate
300g sweetened condensed milk
45g butter
75g salted peanuts

Cut the chocolate into small pieces.

Line a small baking tray (approx 20cm) with cling film.

Melt the butter and condensed milk in a saucepan.

Add the chocolate and stir gently over slow heat until melted but not boiling.

Mix in the peanuts, pour into the baking tray and leave to cool in fridge for 2 hrs.

Cut the fudge into bite-size pieces and enjoy.

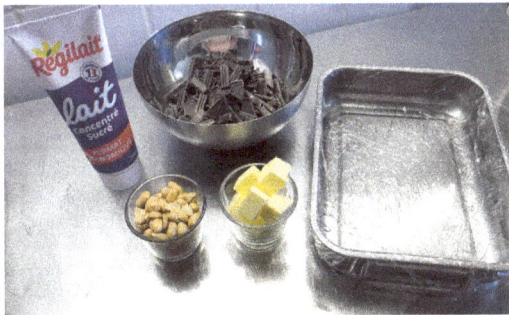

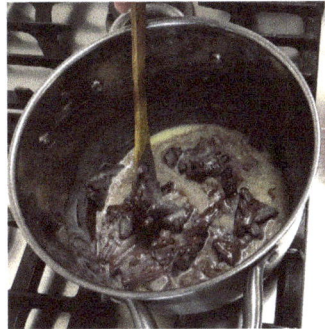

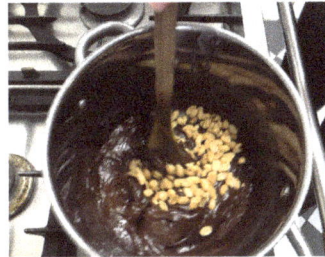

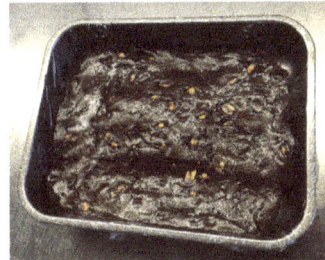

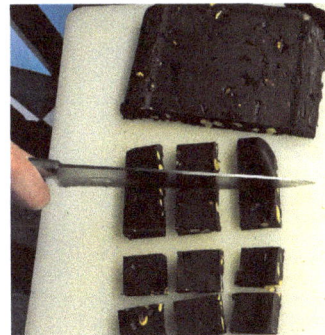

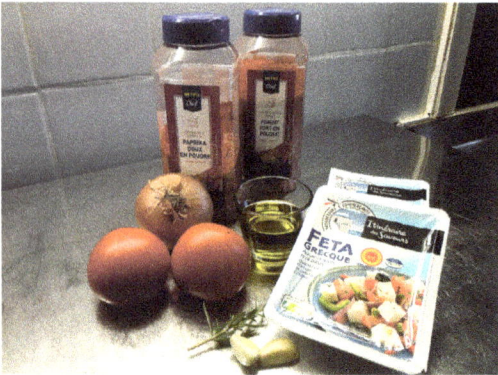

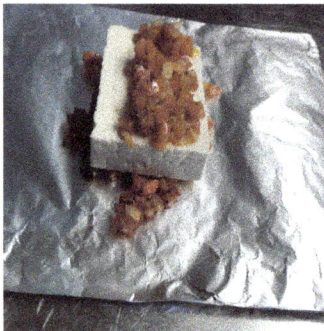

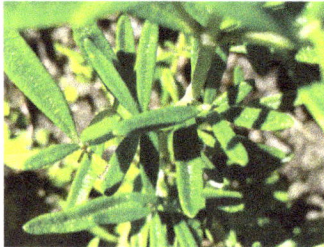

Oven-baked feta

2 blocks of feta cheese
1 onion
2 garlic cloves
2 ripe tomatoes
Rosemary
Sweet paprika powder or hot chilli powder
Olive oil
Salt and pepper
2 pieces of metal foil

Preheat your oven to 220°C or light your BBQ.

Chop the onion, garlic and tomatoes into
small pieces. Chop the rosemary.

Mix everything together well with oilive oil,
herbs and spices, adding a liitle salt
and pepper.

Place 1/4 of the tomato mix on each sheet
of foil, put a block of feta on top of it and
cover with the remaining tomato salsa.

Wrap the feasts into little parcels
and bake in the oven for approx 12 min.

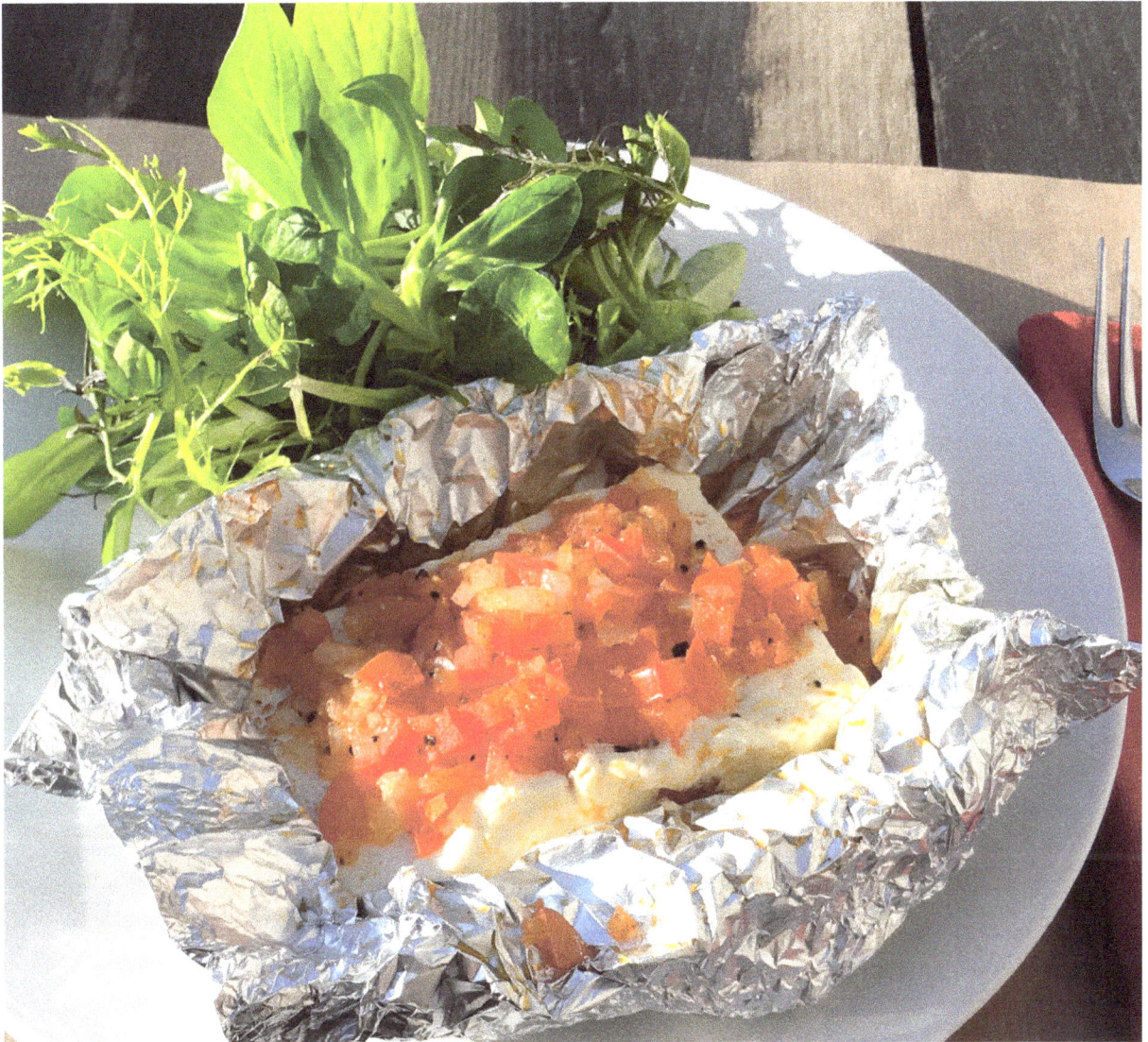

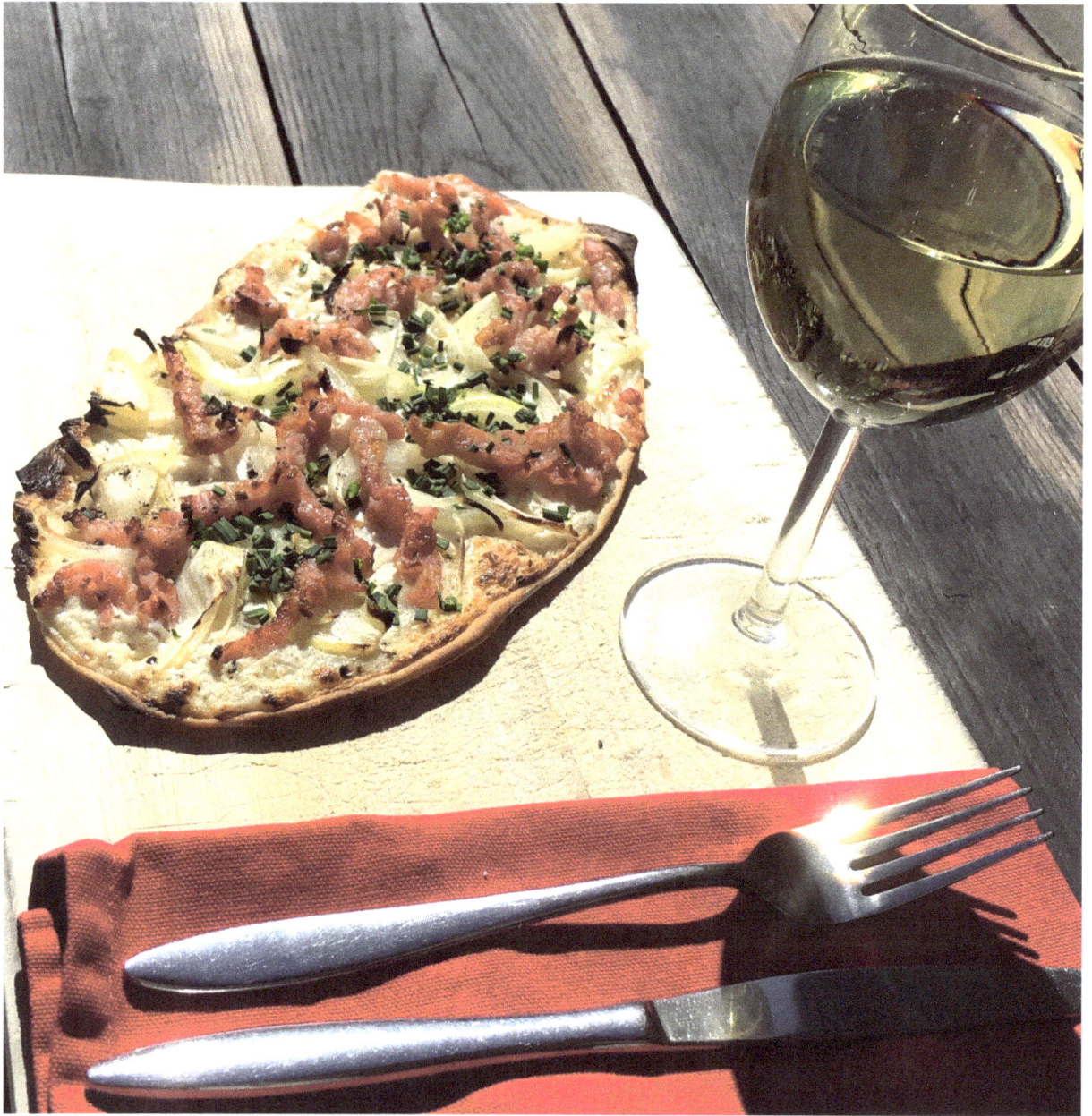

Flammekueche
(serves 3-4)

200g flour
100ml lukewarm water
2 tsp oil
Salt
200g crème fraiche
200g onions cut in stripes
150g bacon pieces
Salt, pepper and nutmeg

Mix the flour, water and a little salt and
form into a smooth pastry. Wrap it in cling film and
leave to rest in the fridge for 30 min.

Season the crème fraiche with a little salt,
pepper and nutmeg.

Preheat your oven to 250°C with a large flat
baking tray in the oven.

Cut the pastry in 4 equal pieces and roll them out
very thin. Spread crème fraiche on each piece
and place the bacon pieces and onion on top.

Bake the flammküchen on the hot baking tray
for 12 min or until crispy.

Goes very well with a cold glass
of dry white wine.

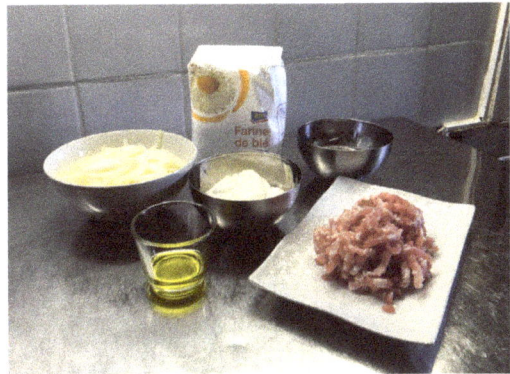

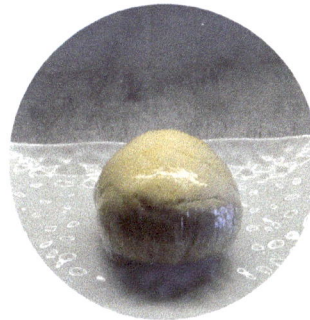

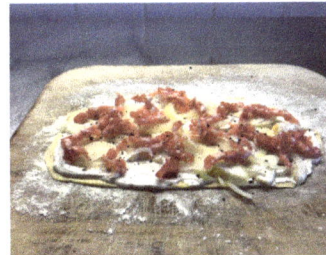

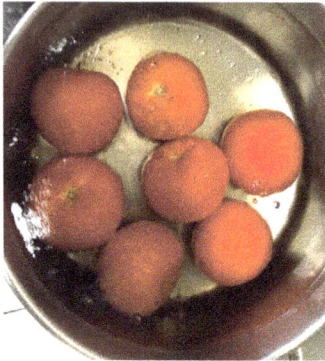

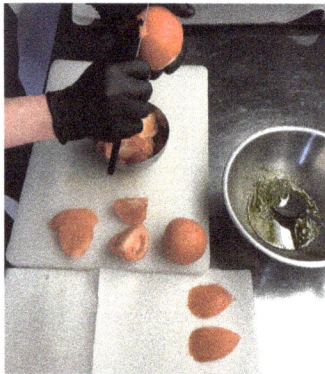

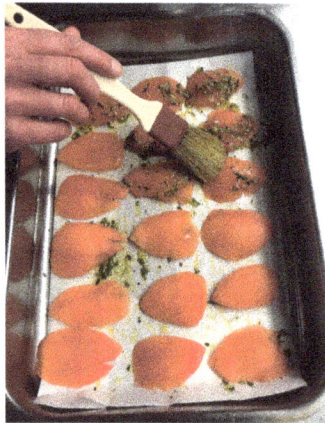

Dried tomatoes
(for tomorrow's recipe)

7 tomatoes
Rosemary, finely chopped
2 cloves of garlic, chopped
50ml olive oil
1 tsp sugar
1 tsp salt

Preheat your oven to 130°C.

Plunge the tomatoes into boiling water
for a few seconds and transfer immediately
into icy cold water to loosen their skin.

Peel the skin off the tomatoes.
Remove seeds and cut in quarters.

Mix the oil, garlic, rosemary, salt and
sugar together well.

Place the quartered tomatoes on a baking tray
lined with baking paper, and brush them with
the oil mixture.

Leave the tomatoes in the oven for 2 1/2 hrs,
turning them every 30 min. Leave the oven door
slightly open for steam to escape.

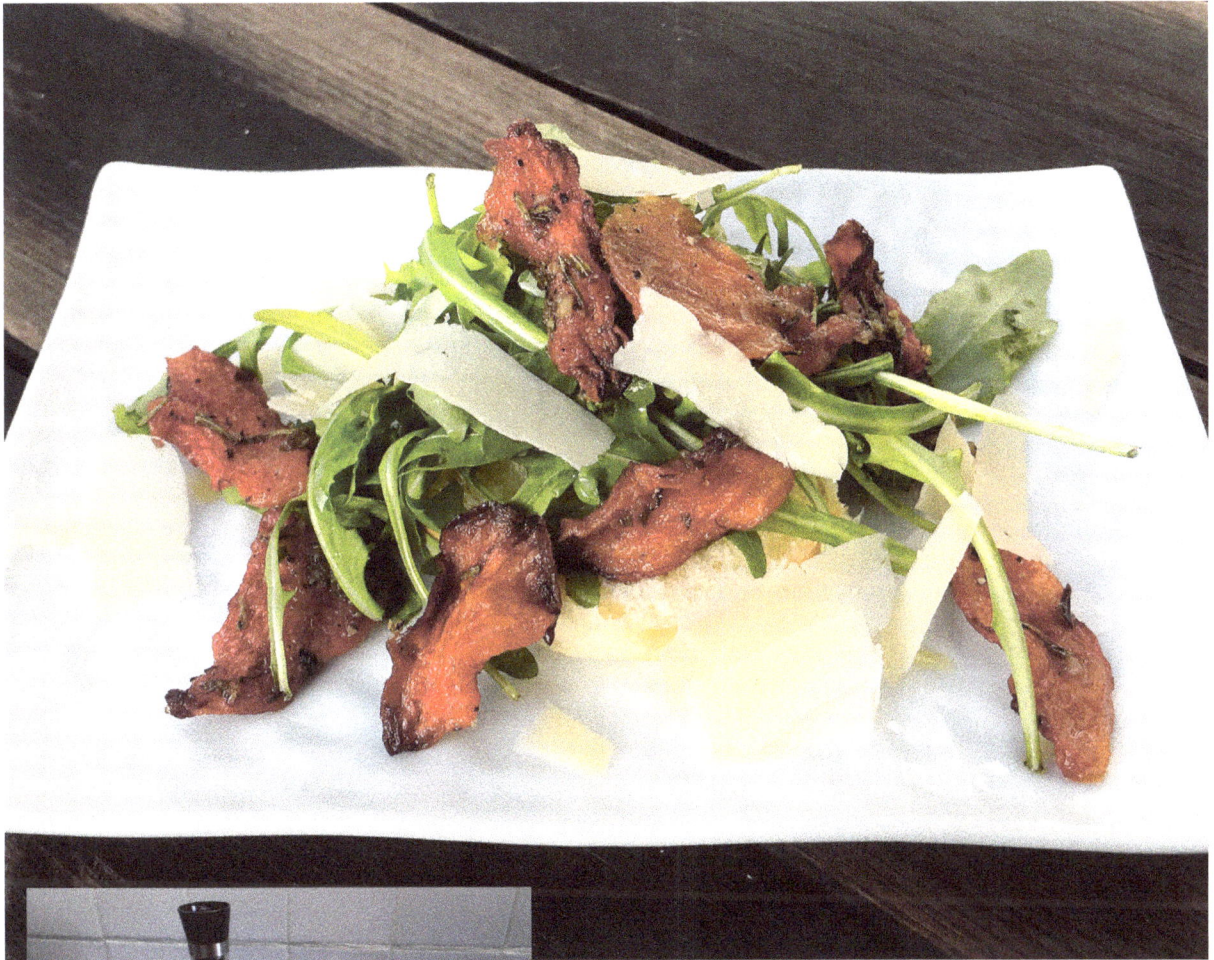

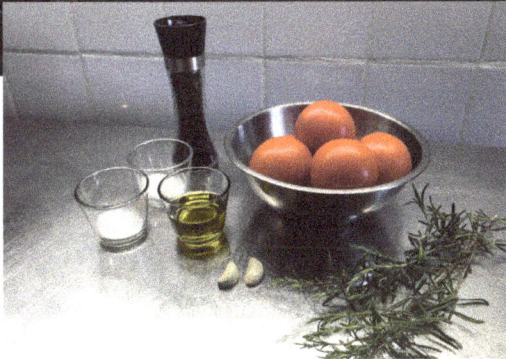

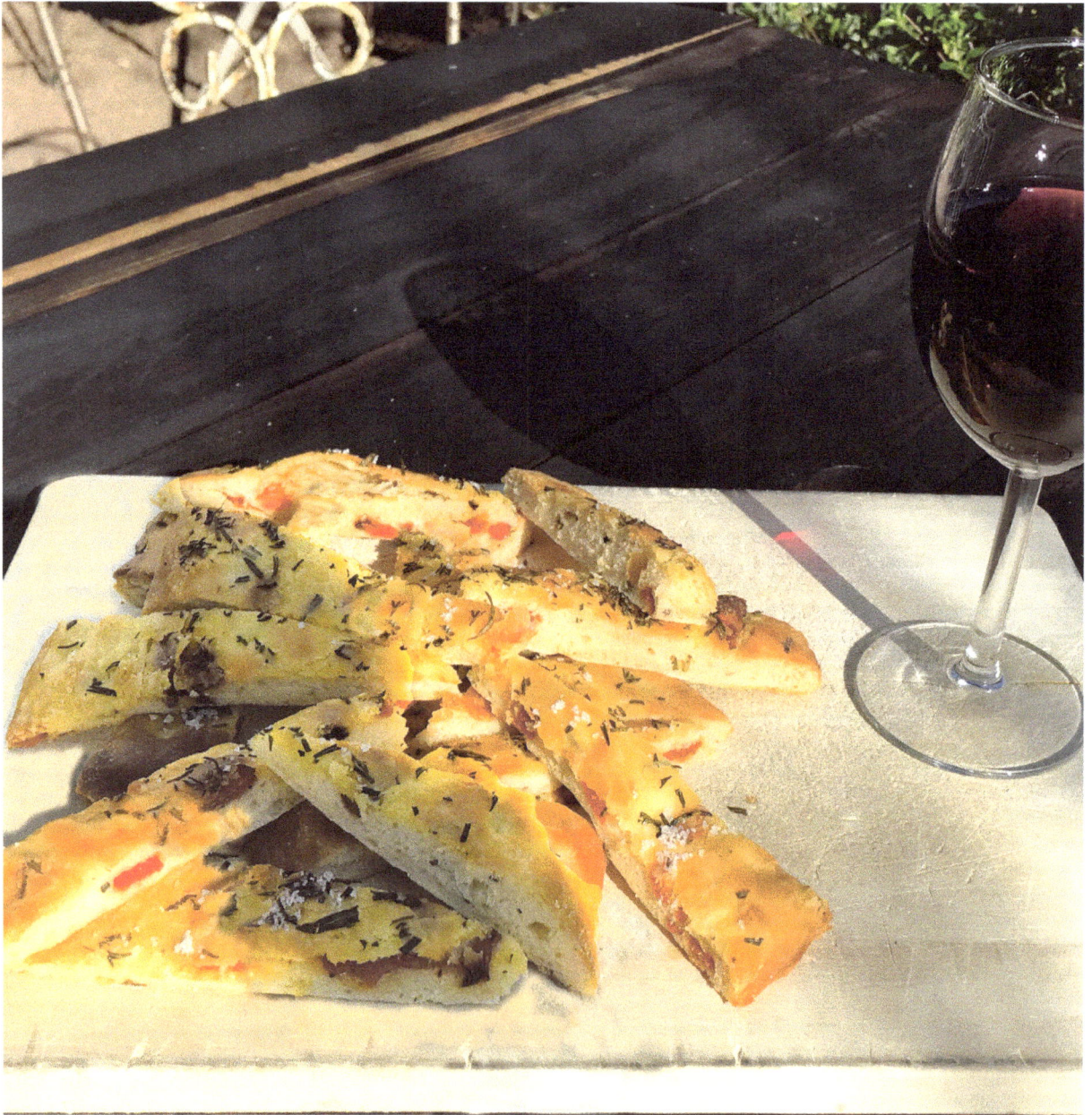

Dried tomato focaccia

250g flour
2 tsp yeast
1/2 tsp salt
Chopped rosemary (about 8 branches)
7–8 tbsp olive oil
150ml water
10 dried tomatoes, diced
Fleur de sel

Preheat your oven to 200°C.

Mix the yeast with lukewarm water.

Prepare a dough with the flour, the water/yeast mixture, half the rosemary, salt and 2 tbsp of olive oil.

Let it rise for 30 min.

Knead the dough and roll it out to about 20x30cm.

With your finger tips, make small holes in the dough. Leave to rest for another 10 min.

Brush it with 3–4 tbsp olive oil and sprinkle with fleur de sel and the rest of the rosemary.

Spray a little water on top. Bake for 12–15 min.

When cooked, brush the top with olive oil and leave to cool.

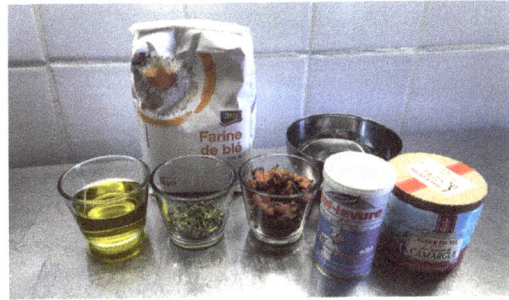

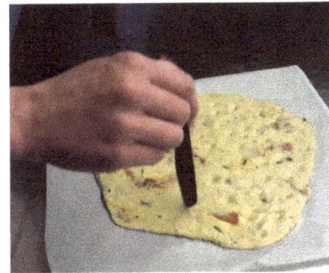

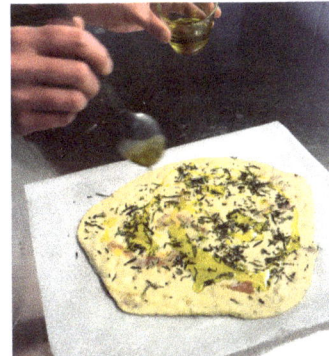

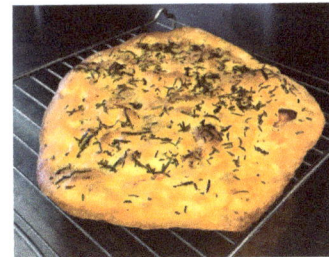

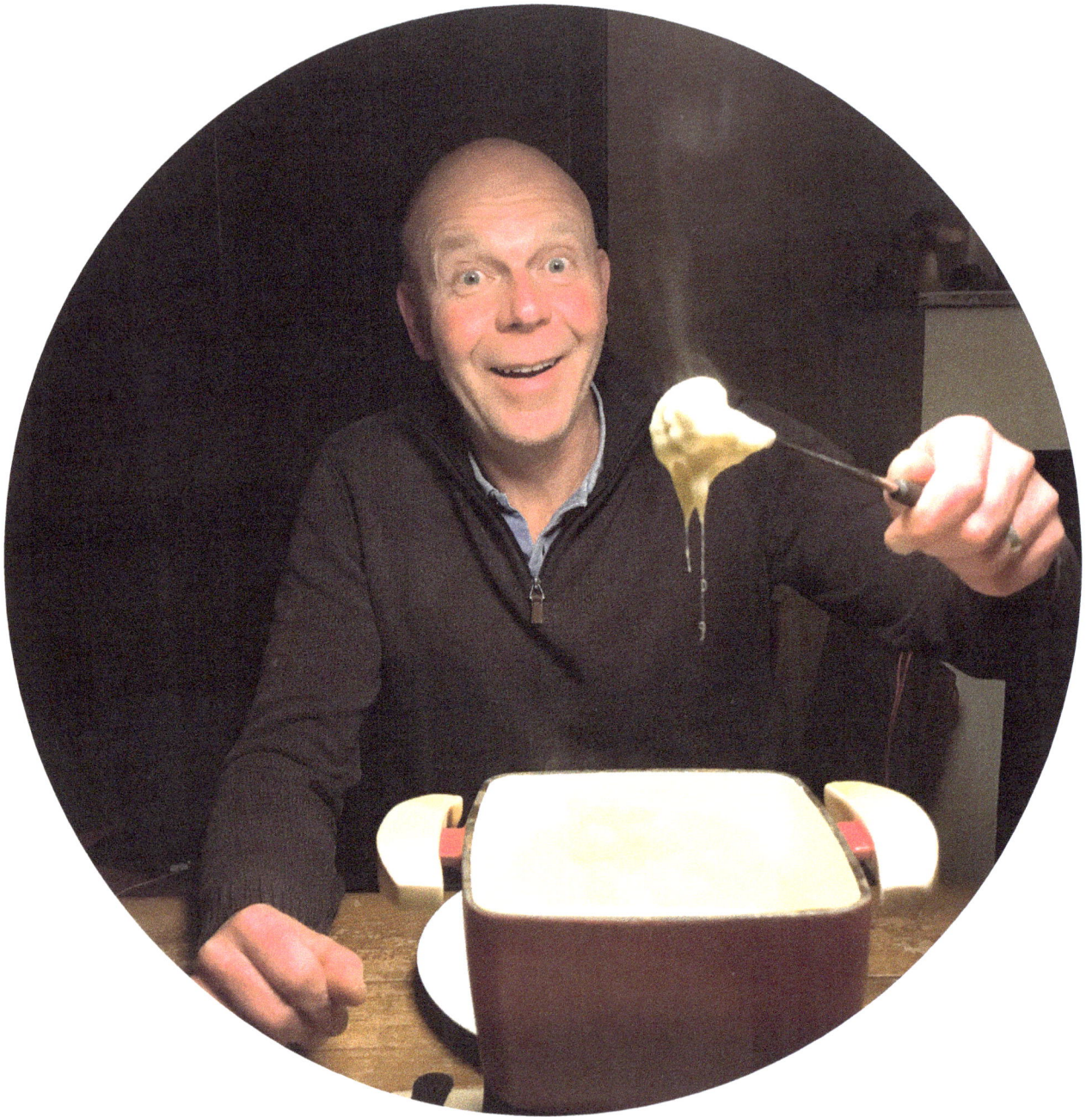

Three-cheese fondue
(serves 4)

400g grated emmental cheese
200g grated Gruyere cheese
200g of grated comté cheese
3 cloves of garlic
4 tsp cornstarch
1 tsp lemon juice
350ml white wine
Pepper
Nutmeg
1 tbsp of kirsch (optional)
Crusty bread cut in pieces

Rub the inside of the fondue pot with the garlic.

Pour in the white wine and heat to
just before boiling point.

Mix the three cheeses and the cornstarch
in a bowl and add little by little to
the hot wine, stirring constantly.

Season with pepper, nutmeg and kirsch.

Et voilà, it's ready to eat!

Dip the bread pieces into the hot fondue.

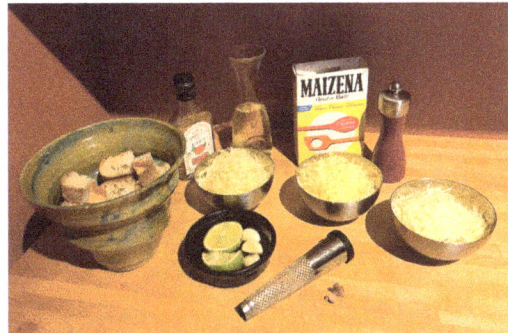

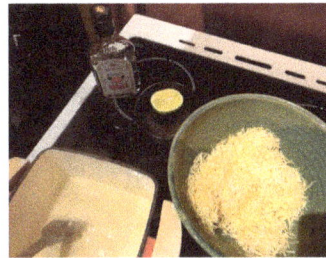

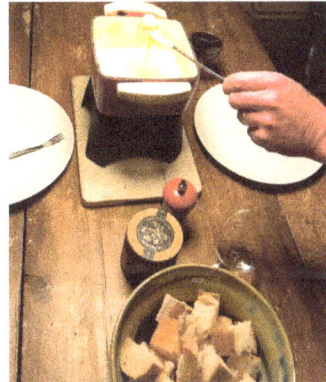

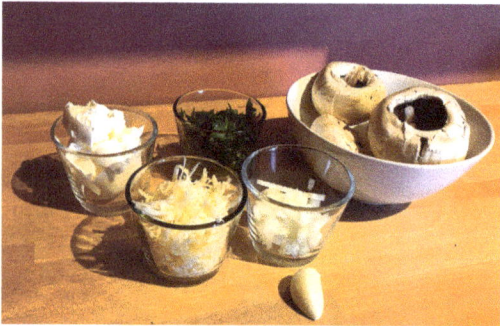

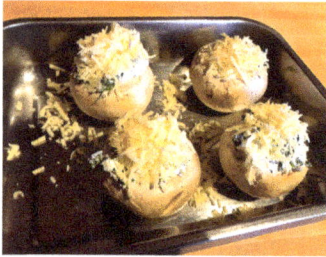

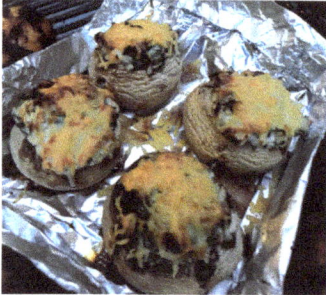

Stuffed mushrooms

4 large mushrooms
1/2 clove of garlic, minced
1/4 chopped onion
70g cheese spread
50g grated Parmesan cheese
Chopped parsley
Salt, pepper

Heat your BBQ (or oven to 200°C).

Mix the cheese spread with the onion,
garlic and parsley.
Season with salt and pepper.

Remove the stems from the mushrooms.

Stuff the mushroom caps with the cheese spread
mixture. Sprinkle with Parmesan.

Grill for about 10 min.

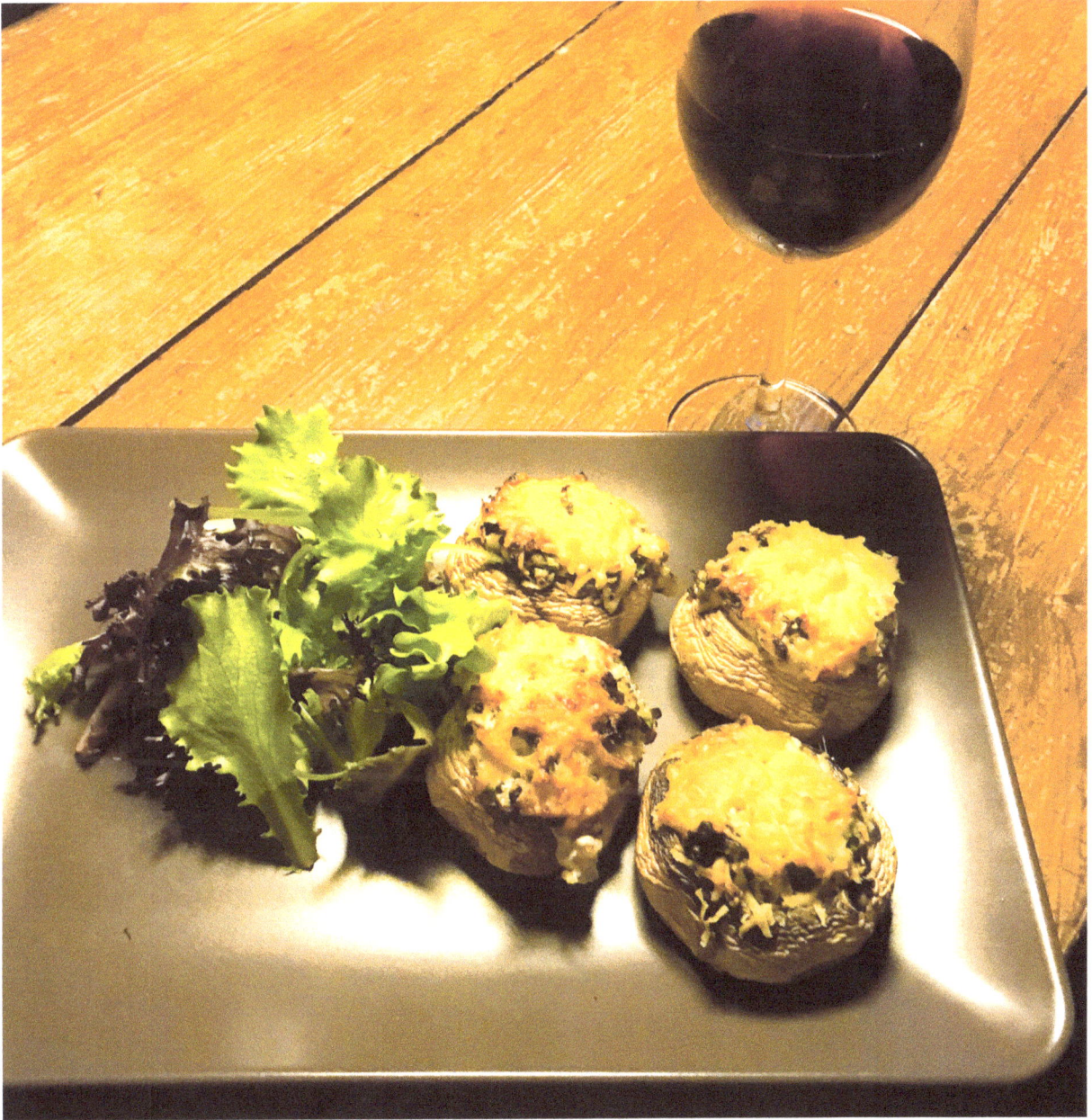

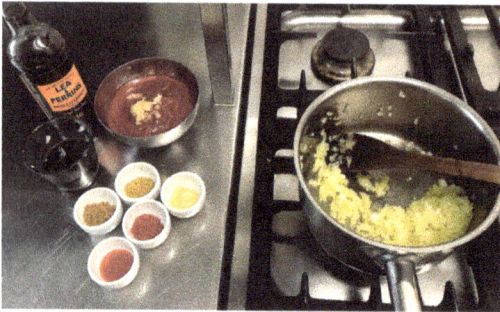

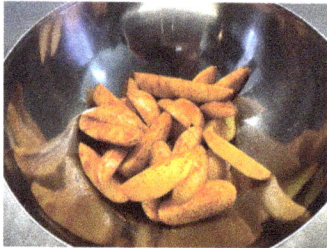

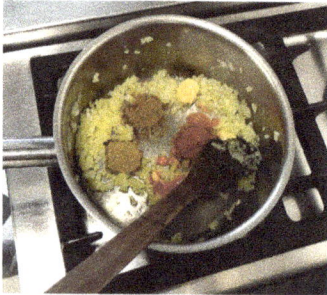

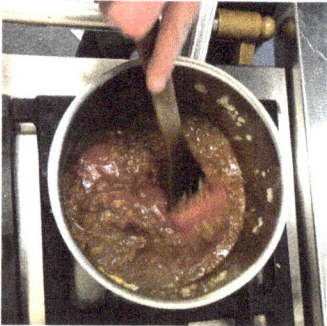

Wedges and BBQ sauce

500g potatoes
2 tbsp oil
1 tsp ground paprika
1 tsp hot pepper powder
Salt, fleur de sel
*
250ml ketchup
330ml Coca Zero
1 chopped onion
1 clove of garlic, chopped
1 tsp mustard
1/4 tsp cumin
1/4 tsp curry powder
2 tsp Worcestershire sauce
1 tbsp sugar
1/2 tsp sriracha sauce (optional)

Preheat your oven to 200°C.

Cut the potatoes into quarters and marinate them with
oil, ground paprika and hot pepper powder.

Bring the Coca Zero to the boil in a saucepan
and let it reduce to approx 80ml.

Brown the onion and garlic in a little oil
in a separate saucepan.

Add the spices, mustard, sriarcha sauce, Worcestershire,
ketchup, sugar and reduced Coke.

Boil gently for 5 min.

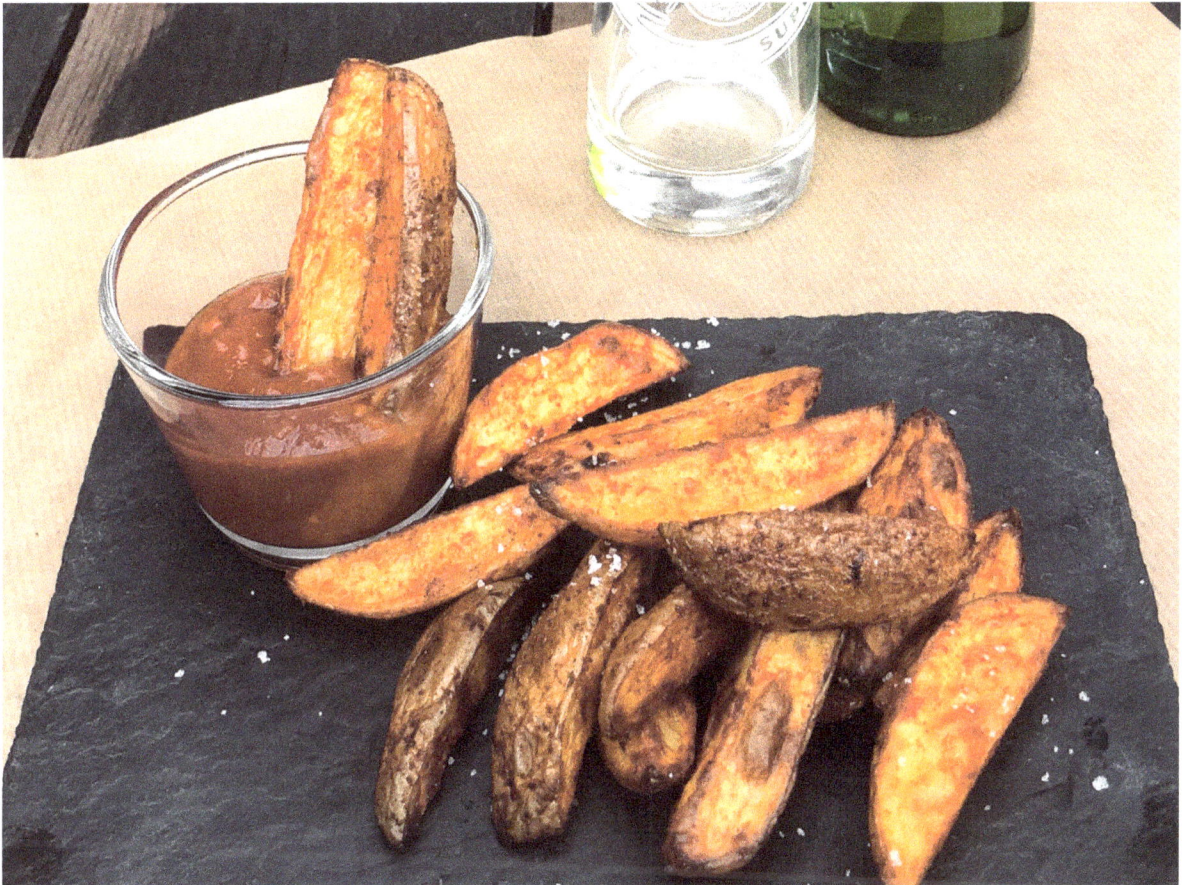

Season with salt and pepper. Leave to cool.

Place the marinated potato wedges on a baking sheet
and bake them for 15 min.

Turn the potatoes over and return to the oven
for about 10 min.

Season with fleur de sel (or salt).

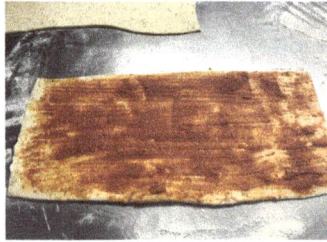

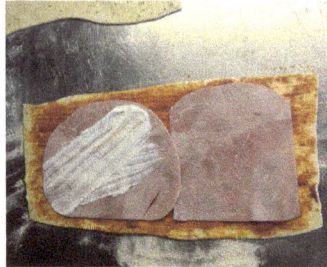

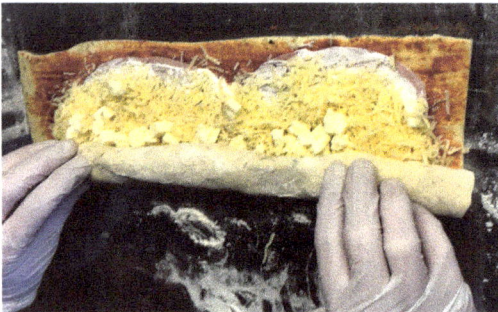

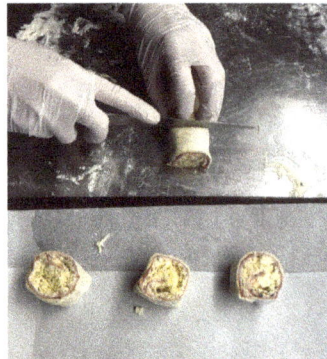

Mini pizza rolls
(makes about 24)

280g flour
150ml lukewarm water
7g dry yeast
1 tsp salt
2 tsp dried oregano
1 tbsp olive oil
*
3 tbsp tomato paste
1 clove of garlic, minced
4 slices of ham
1 ball of mozzarella, cut into small cubes
100g grated cheese
80g crème fraîche
Salt, pepper

Dissolve the yeast in the warm water.
Prepare a dough with the flour, water/yeast, oil, salt
and oregano and let it rise for 30 min.

Preheat your oven to 200°C.

Mix the minced garlic with the tomato paste.

Roll out the dough until it is the size of your baking
sheet. Cut in two equal parts. Spread tomato paste on
one half of the dough, place 2 slices of ham on top, then
spread on the crème fraîche and sprinkle with the grated
cheese and mozzarella. Repeat with the other half.
Roll up the dough and cut into small slices.
Leave to rise for another 10 min.

Bake for about 12 min.

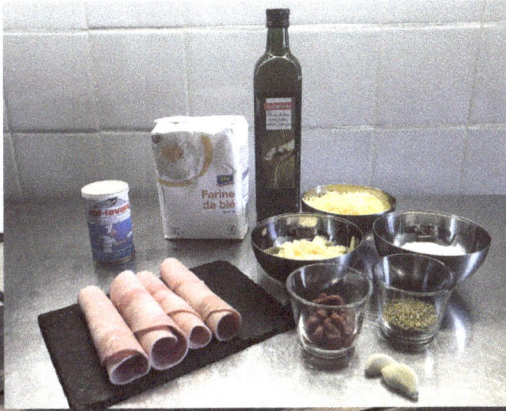

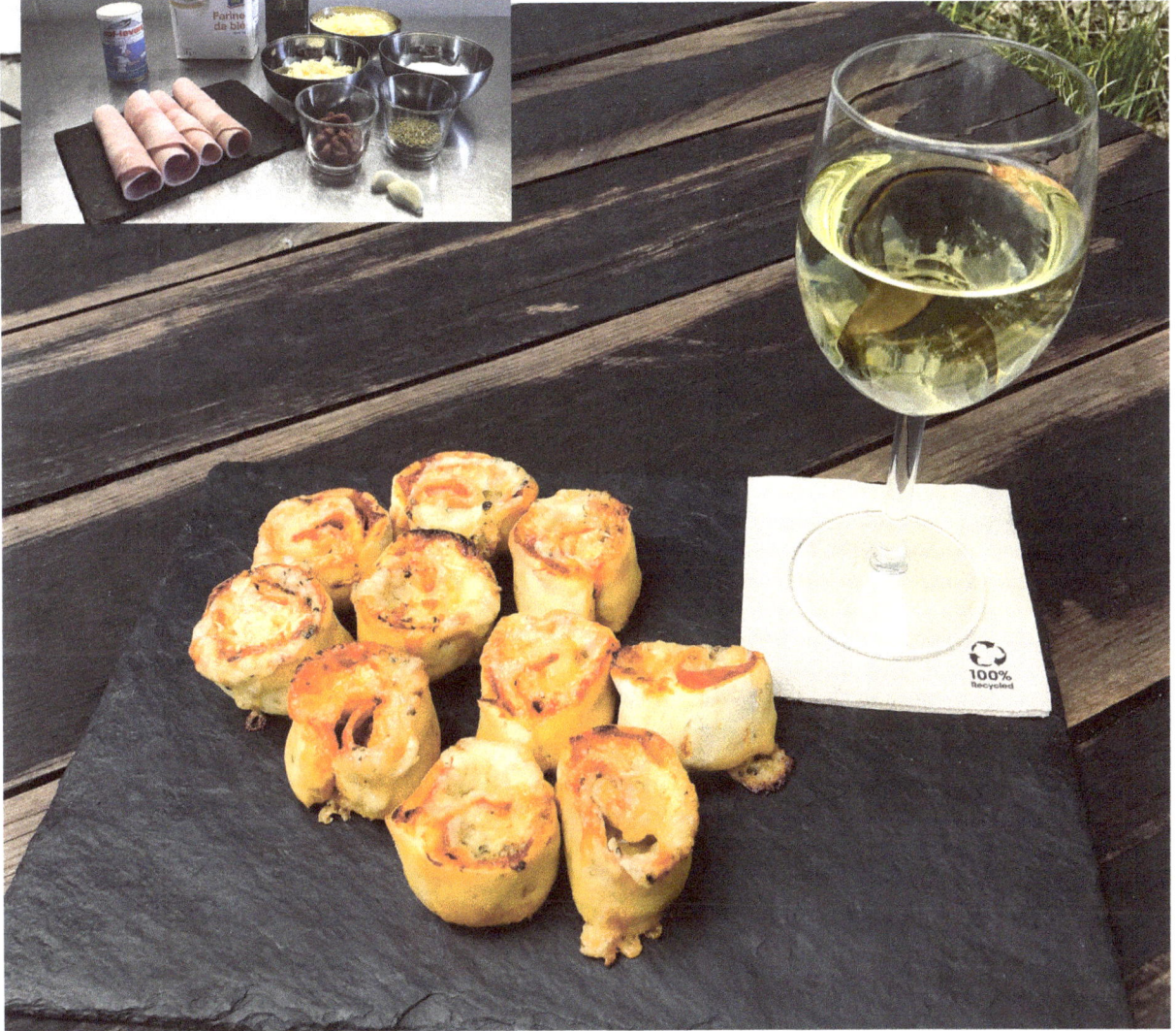

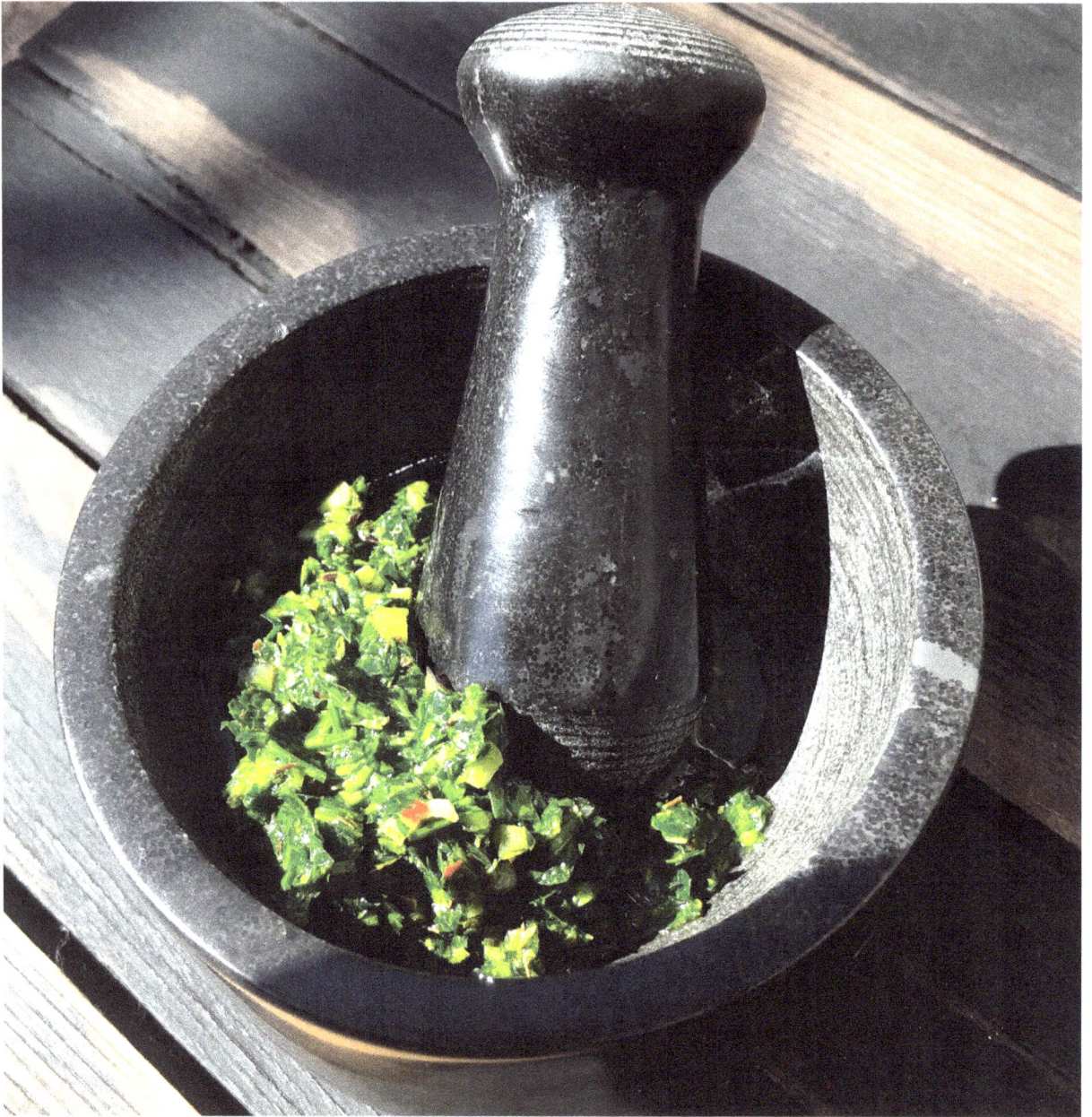

Chimichurri
*(super good with grilled meats,
potatoes or vegetables)*

2 bunches parsley
1 red onion
2 cloves of garlic
Juice of a lime
1/2 tsp chilli flakes
1 tsp dried oregano
1 tsp dried thyme
100ml olive oil
Fleur de sel, pepper

Chop the parsley, onion and garlic.

Crush all the ingredients in a mortar using a pestle
or put them in a blender.

Season with fleur de sel and pepper.

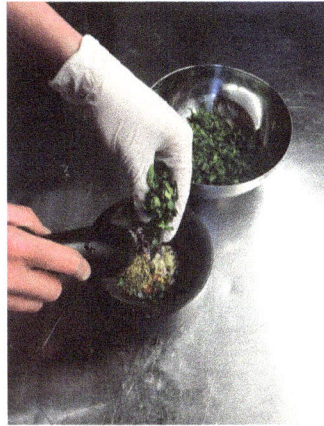

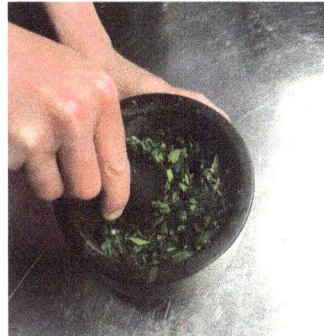

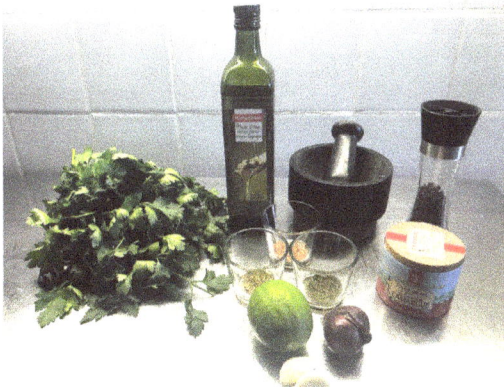

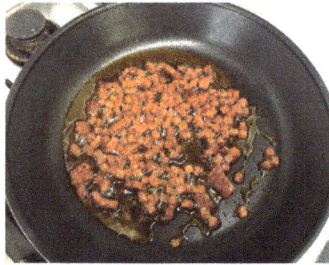

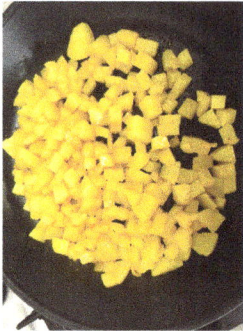

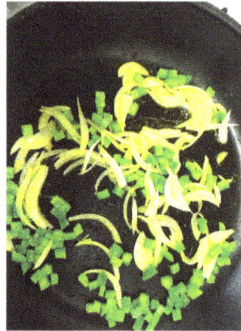

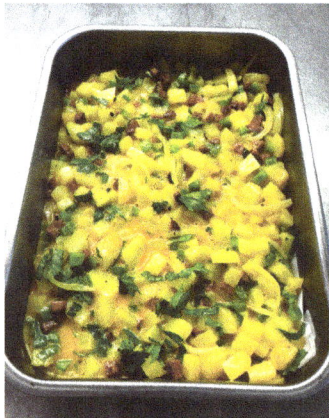

Potato tortilla with chorizo

(makes 24 pieces)

500g potatoes
125g chorizo, diced
4 eggs
1/2 onion, cut into thin strips
1/4 green pepper, finely diced
Salt, pepper

Cook the potatoes 'al dente' and leave to cool.

Preheat your oven to 160°C.

Peel the potatoes and cut them into small cubes.

Heat a little olive oil in a pan and brown the chorizo.
Remove the chorizo and brown the dice potatoes
in the same pan. Remove and mix with the chorizo.

Brown the onion strips and diced green pepper.
Mix in the potatoes and the chorizo.

Break the eggs and season them with salt
and pepper. Mix everything together.

Cover a baking sheet with baking paper
and spread the mixture on it.

Bake for about 12–15 min.

Cut into small pieces.

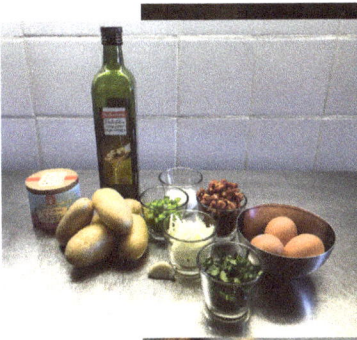

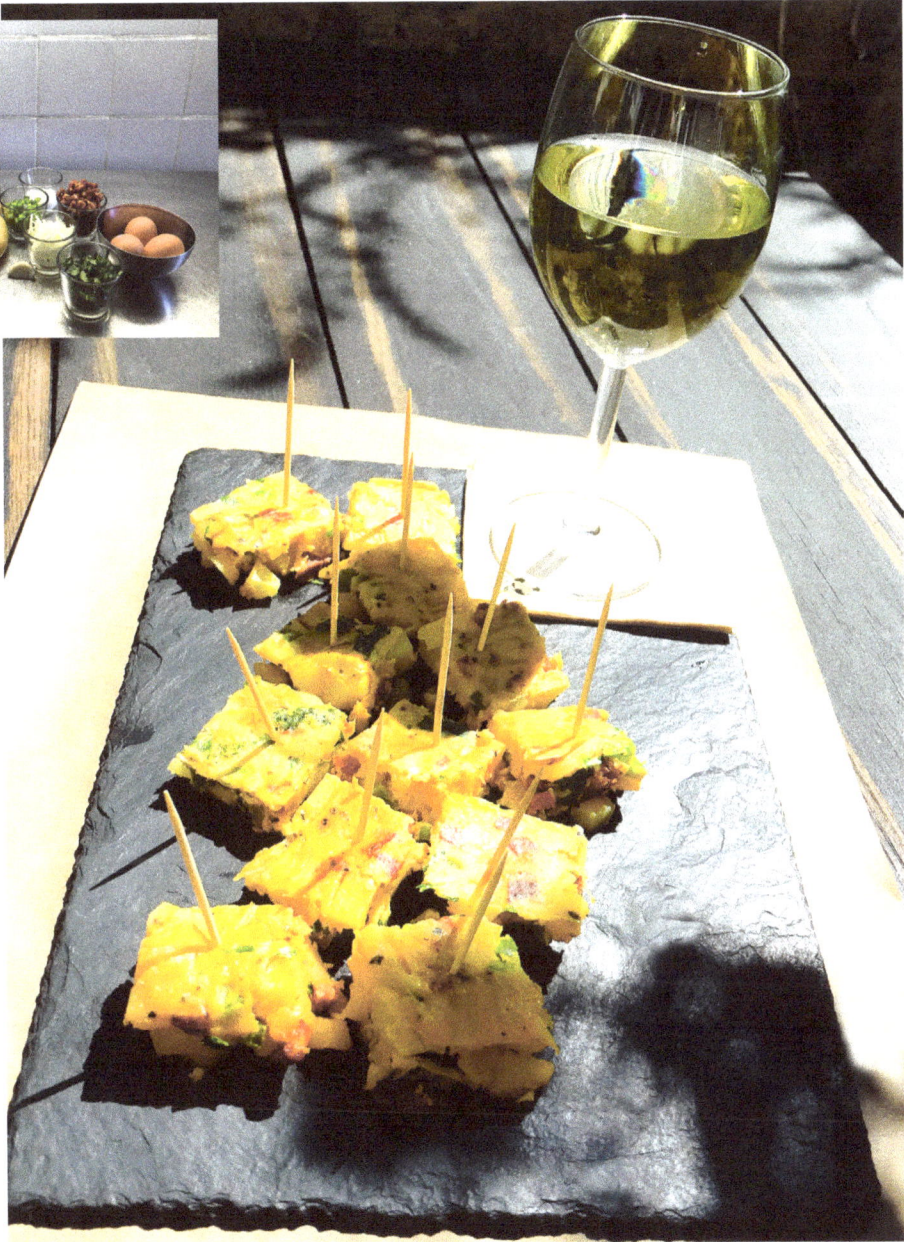

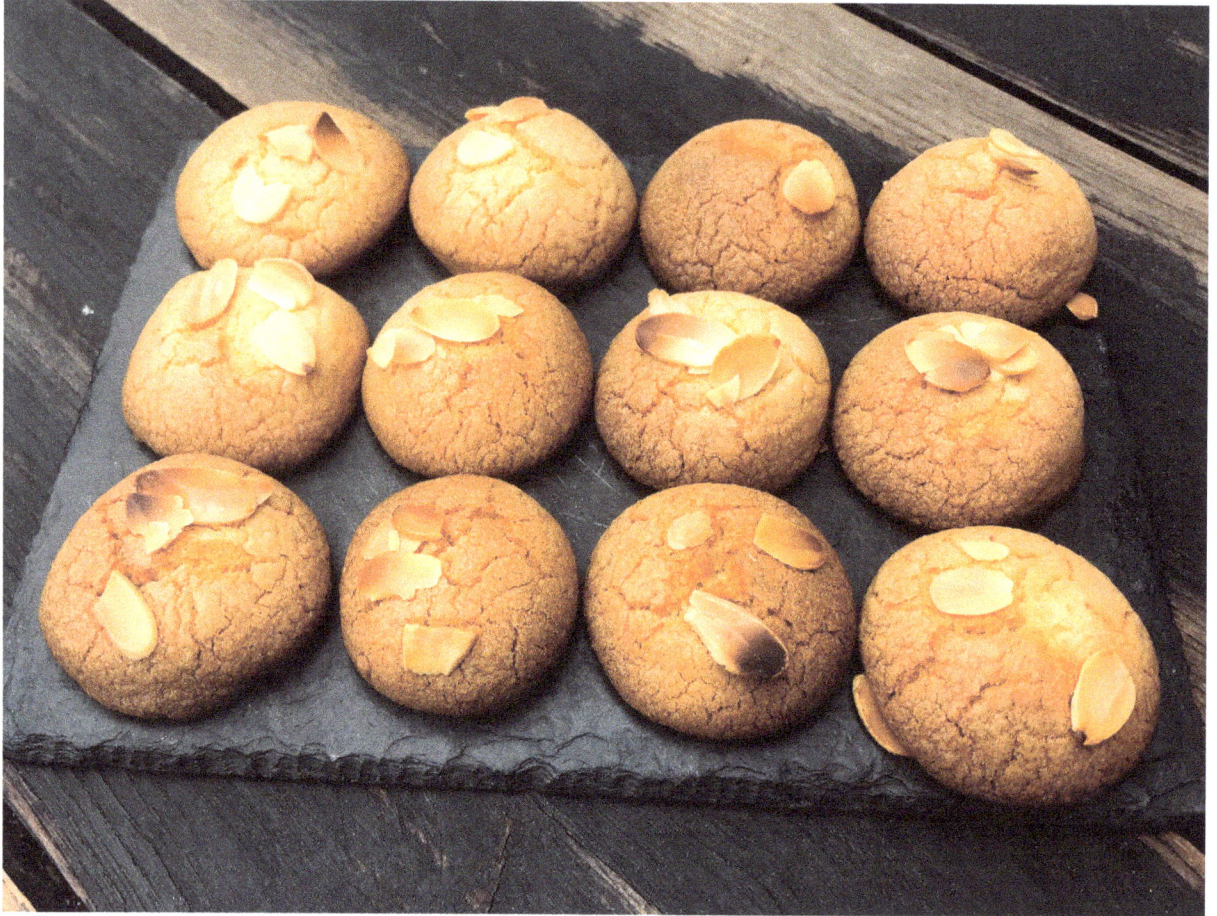

Nankhatai
(Indian cookies)

150g flour
3 tbsp chick pea flour
50g semolina
1/2 tsp baking powder
135g icing sugar
150g butter
2 tbsp yogurt
15g almonds
1 tsp ground cardamom

Preheat your oven to 180°C.

Mix the flour, semolina and baking powder.

Cream the butter with the icing sugar.

Add the yogurt.

Add the dry ingredients and knead until you obtain
a smooth paste. Leave it to rest for 10 min.

Form small balls and place them on your baking sheet.

Garnish with almonds and cook for about 10–12 min.

Allow cookies to cool before serving.

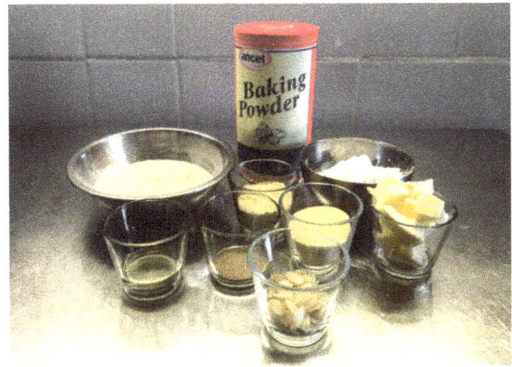

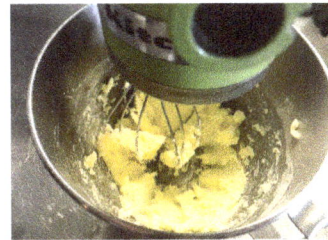

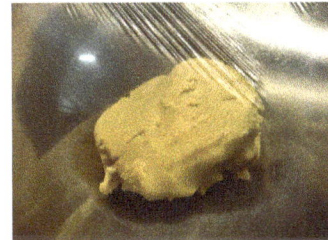

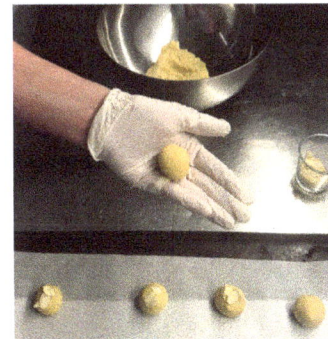

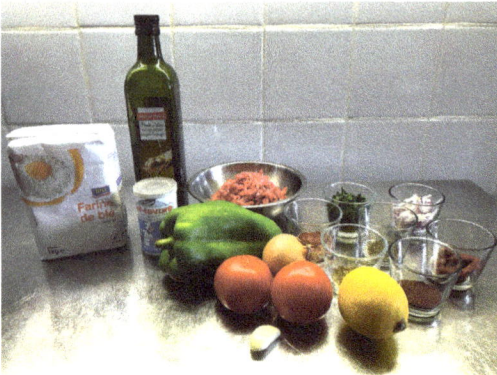

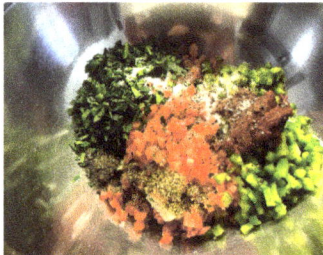

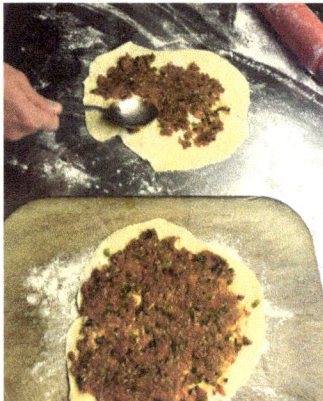

Lahmacun
(makes 7 pieces)

Dough:
400g flour
250ml lukewarm water
20ml olive oil
7g salt
4g dry yeast
1/2 tsp sugar

*

250g minced meat (beef or lamb)
2 tomatoes
1/2 green pepper
Parsley
1 onion
1 clove of garlic
1 tbsp harissa puree
1 tbsp tomato paste
1/4 tbsp dried thyme
1/4 tbsp dried oregano
Olive oil
Salt and pepper

*

Toppings:
Diced tomatoes, thinly sliced red onions,
parsley, lemon, sumac (optional)

Prepare a dough and leave it to rise for 45 min.
Preheat your oven to 230°C (with the baking tray
in the oven).

Cut all the vegetables into very small cubes.

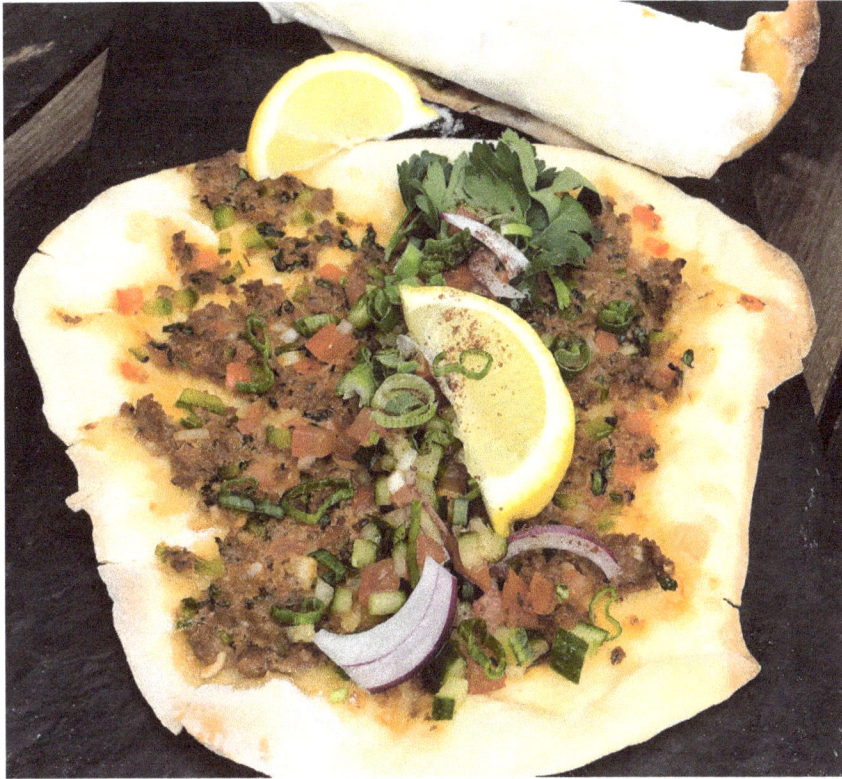

Mix all the ingredients well with minced meat.

Season with salt, pepper and olive oil.

Divide the dough into small balls of about 90g.

Roll out the dough very thinly and spread
2 tbsp of the minced meat mixture
on to the dough.

Put it on the baking tray and bake
for about 5 min.

When the first lahmacun is ready, place it on a
plate and cover it with a kitchen towel.

Continue to cook the lahmacuns. Place the
second on top of the first (meat on meat,
dough on dough).

Cover with cling film (or cooking foil)
for a few minutes.

Garnish your lahmacuns with the toppings,
roll them up and enjoy.

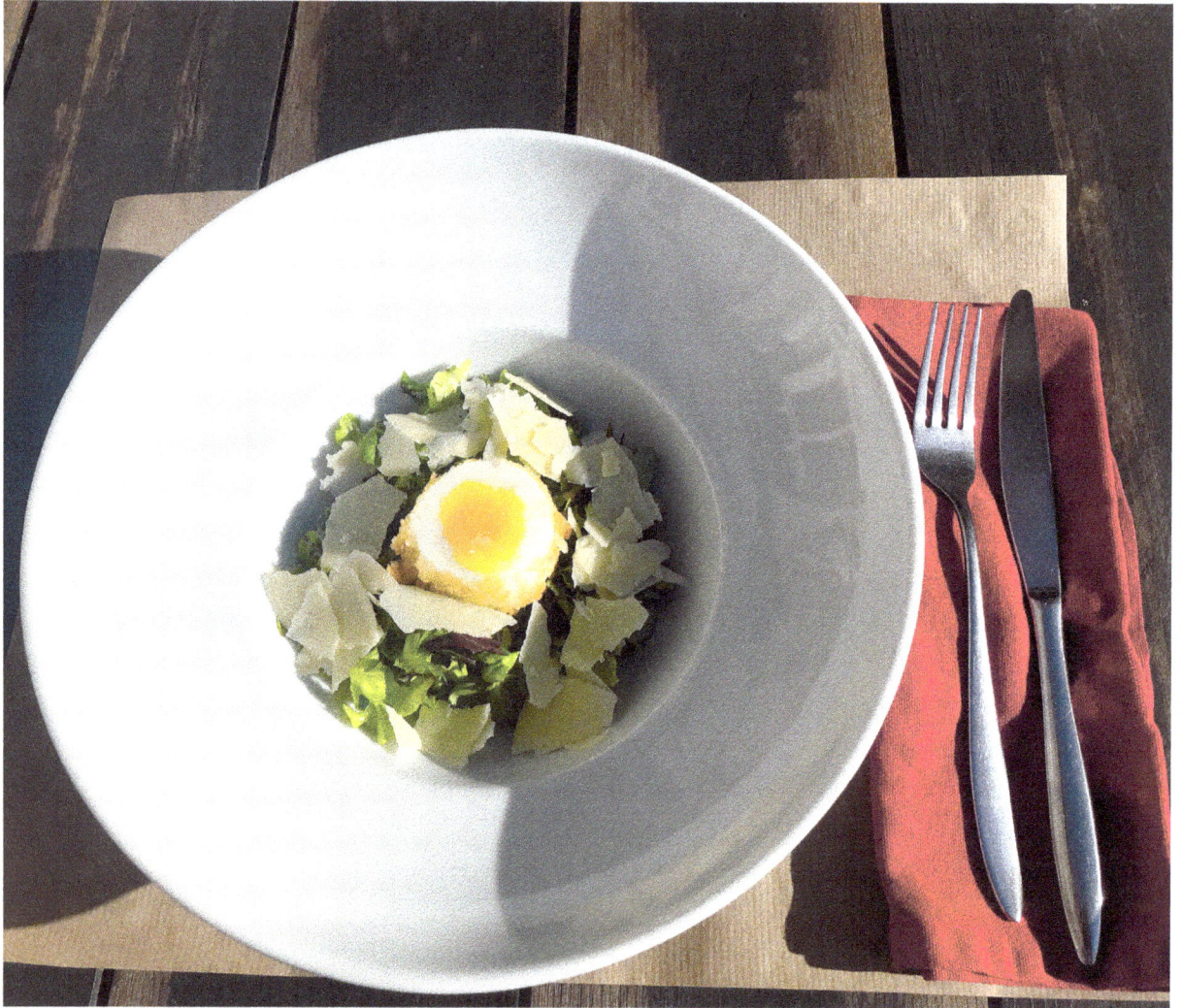

Crumbed eggs

3 eggs
Flour
Panko or breadcrumbs
Frying oil
Salt, pepper
Salad greens
Parmesan cheese

In a saucepan, bring water to the boil.
Cook 2 eggs for 5 min and 30 sec. Cool them down
immediately in icy water.

Carefully peel the eggs.

Heat a little frying oil in a saucepan.

Break the third egg into a bowl and beat with a fork.
Turn the boiled eggs in the flour, then in the
beaten egg and finally in the breadcrumbs.

Drop the breaded eggs in the hot frying oil for
about 1 min or until golden brown.

Season with salt and pepper.

Serve with a fresh garden salad and
grated Parmesan.

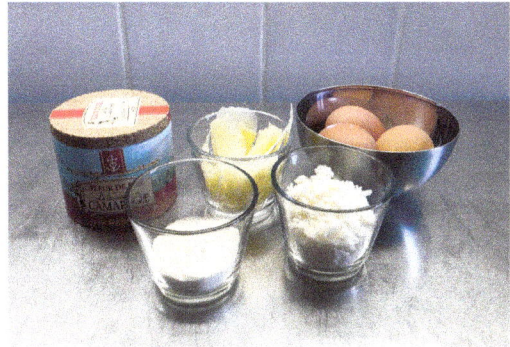

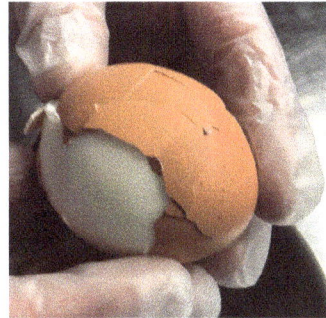

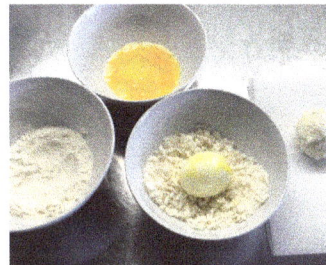

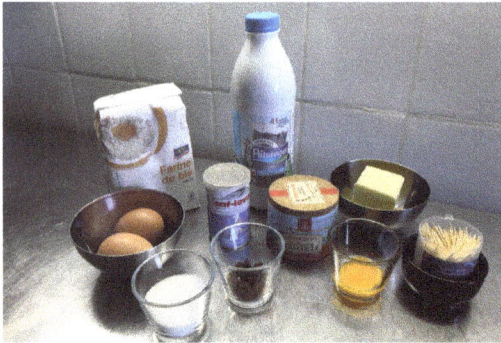

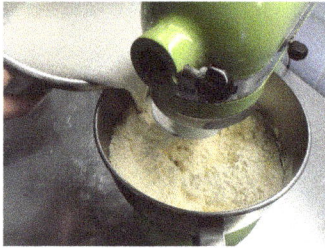

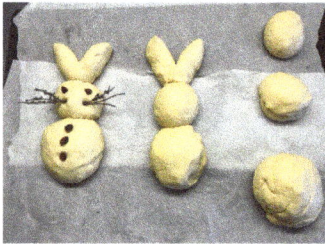

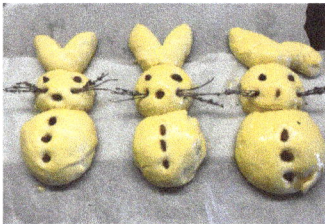

Easter bunnies

1kg of flour
500ml lukewarm milk
4 tsp dry yeast
50g sugar
150g butter, melted
2 eggs

For decoration:
1 egg yolk, raisins, branches of thyme.

Dissolve the yeast and sugar in the lukewarm milk.

Combine the flour and salt in a bowl and add
the butter, eggs and milk mixture.
Prepare a dough and leave it to rise for 1 hr.

Preheat your oven to 200°C.

Cut the dough into nine parts; three big and six small.

Match the three rabbits according to the picture.
Use the raisins for the eyes and belly buttons;
the branches of thyme are perfect
for the whiskers.

Leave to rest for 30 min and brush
with the egg yolk.

Bake for 20–25 min.

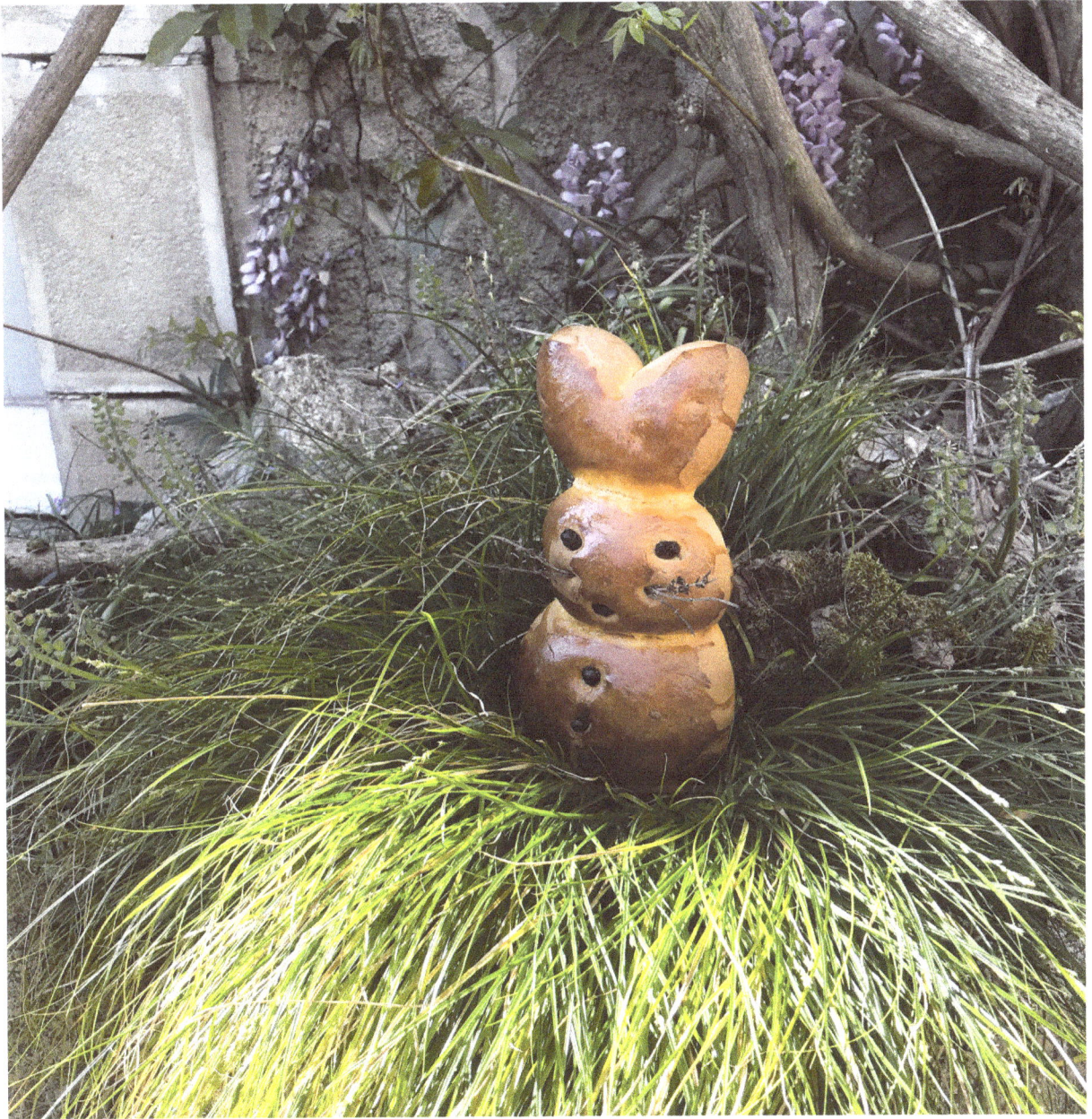

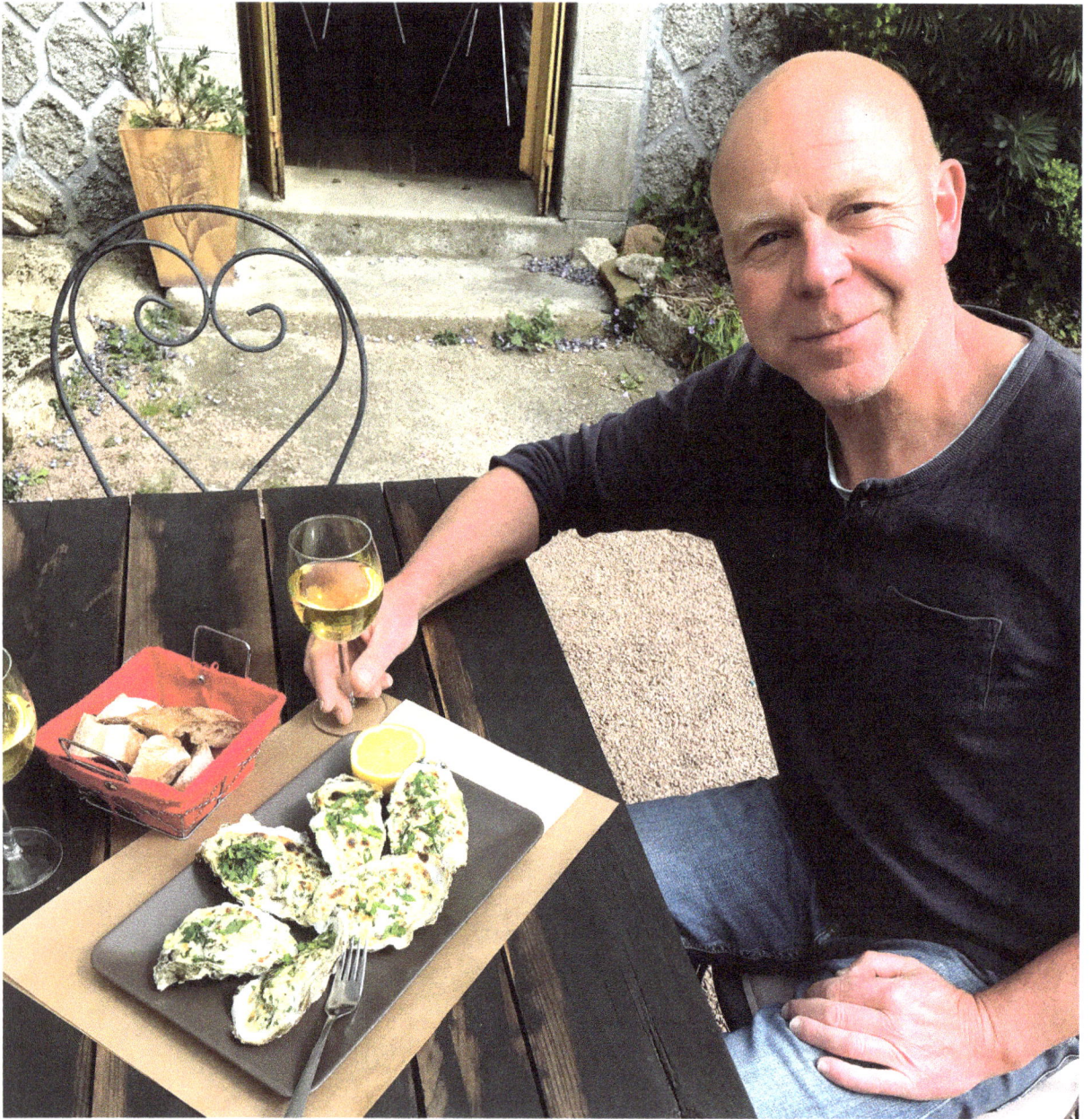

Oysters au gratin

6 oysters No 2
70g crème fraîche
30g grated Parmesan cheese
35ml white wine
1 shallot diced
1 small clove of garlic, diced
Butter
Chopped parsley
Salt, pepper

Remove the oysters from their shells.
Set them aside and clean the shells.
Return the oysters to the shells.

Preheat your oven to 200°C (grill mode).

Melt a little butter in a saucepan and brown
the finely diced shallot and garlic.

Deglaze with the white wine and let it reduce
until there is hardly any liquid left.

Add the crème fraîche, Parmesan and parsley.
Season with salt and pepper.

Place the oysters on a baking sheet and cover
each of them with 1–1 1/2 tbsp of the sauce.

Bake for about 5 min.

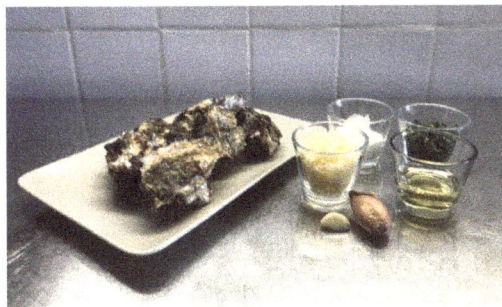

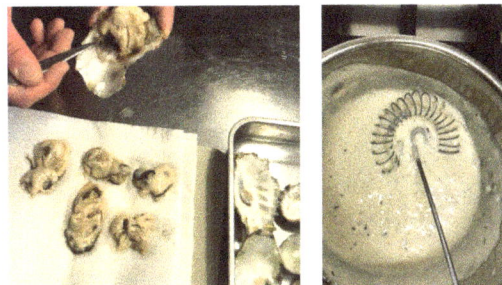

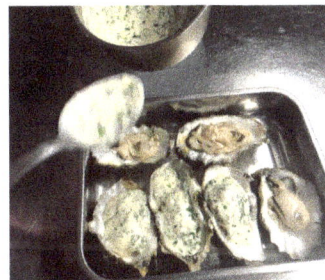

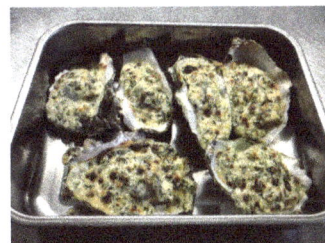

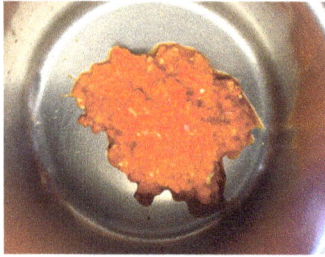

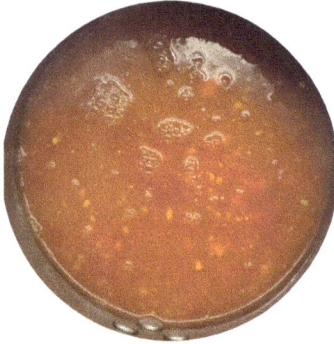

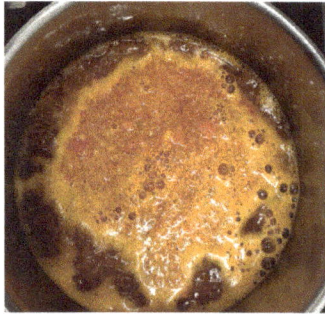

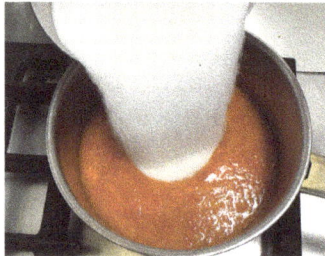

Sweet chilli sauce
(percect with tomorrow's chicken recipe)

120g chopped red peppers
1/4–1/2 chopped Thai chilli (or other chilli)
6 cloves of garlic, chopped
200g sugar
180ml rice vinegar (or white vinegar)
1 tsp salt
80ml water
1 tbsp cornstarch (diluted in 3 tbsp cold water)

Mix the red peppers, chilli and garlic
with 80ml of water.

Pour everything into a saucepan with
the sugar, salt and vinegar.

Bring to a boil and simmer for about 5 min.

Add the cornstarch and simmer for another 1 min.

When your sauce is cool, store it
in a decorative bottle.

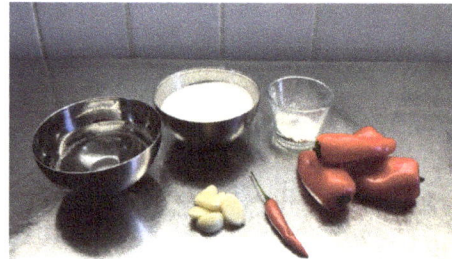

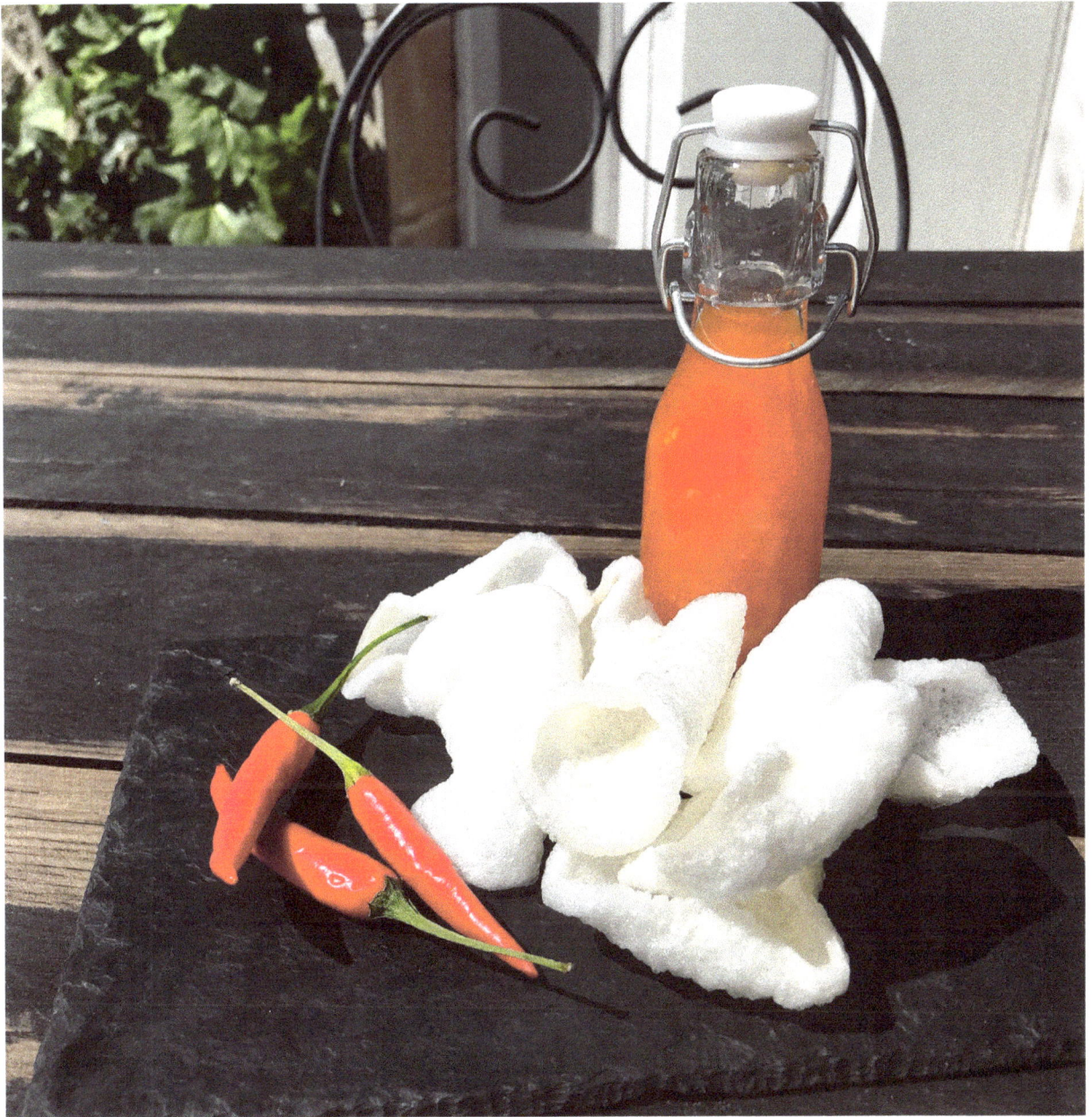

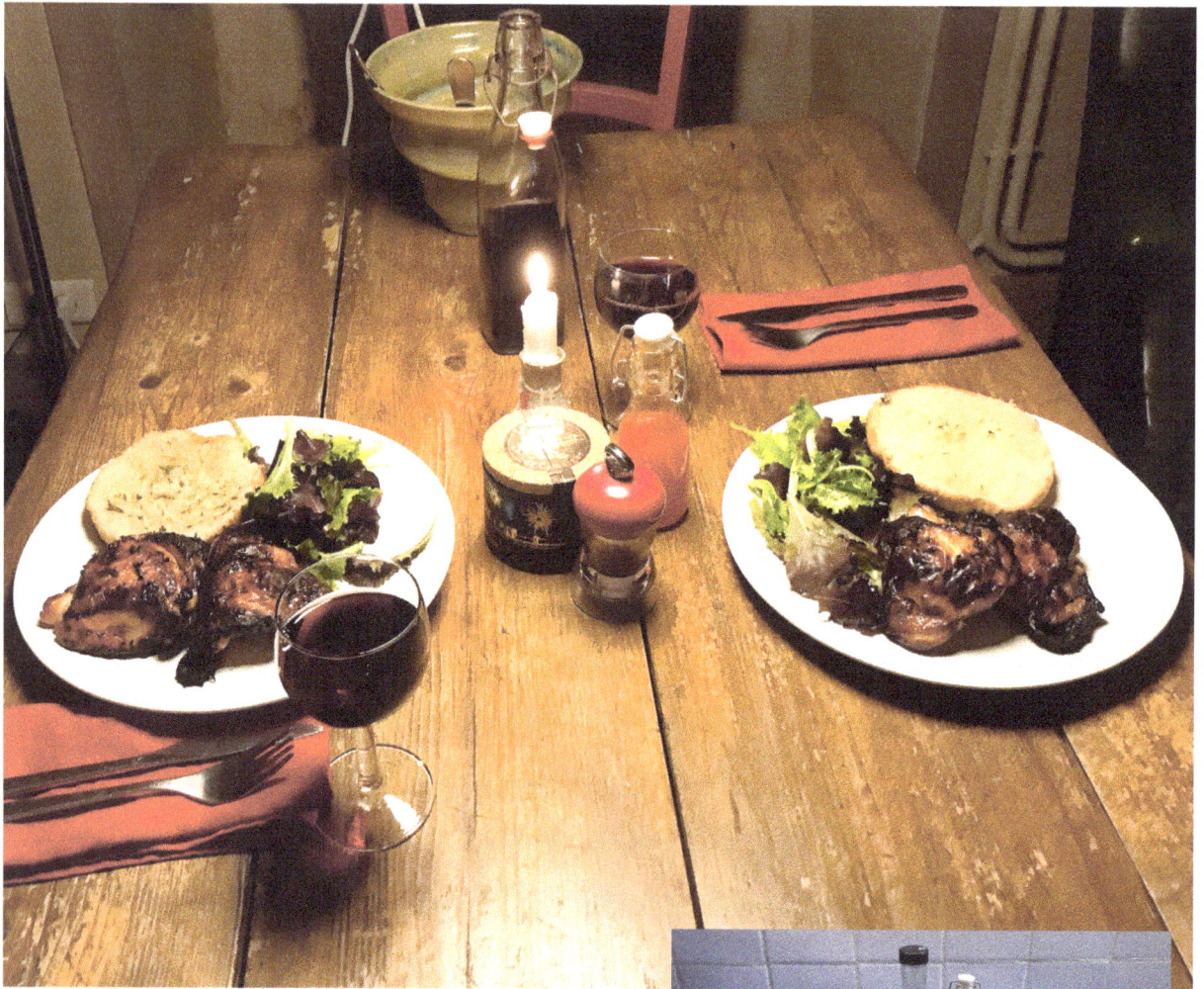

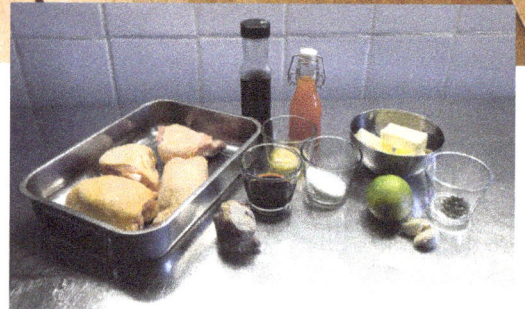

Grilled chicken thighs

Marinade:
4 chicken thighs
Juice of one lime
1 clove of garlic, minced
20g chopped ginger
4 tbsp soy sauce, 1 tbsp honey
2 tbsp sesame oil, 1 tsp sugar
2 tbsp sweet-chilli sauce
*
1 baguette
80g butter
3 cloves of garlic
Zest of a lime
Thyme, salt, pepper

Mix all the ingredients for the marinade and pour onto the chicken thighs. Leave them in the fridge for at least 3 hr, turning them every 30 min.

Mix the butter with the lime zest, chopped garlic and thyme. Season with salt and pepper.

Cut the baguette in half lengthwise. Spread the mixture on it and wrap it in metal baking foil.

Light your BBQ.

Grill the chicken thighs for about 15–20 min.

5 min before the end of cooking, place the wrapped baguette on the BBQ.
Serve with the sweet chilli sauce from yesterday.

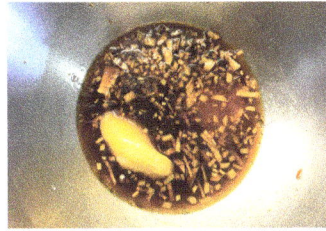

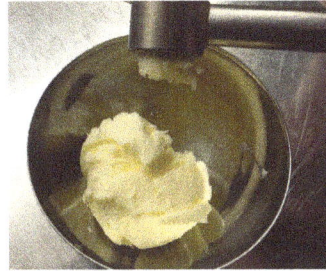

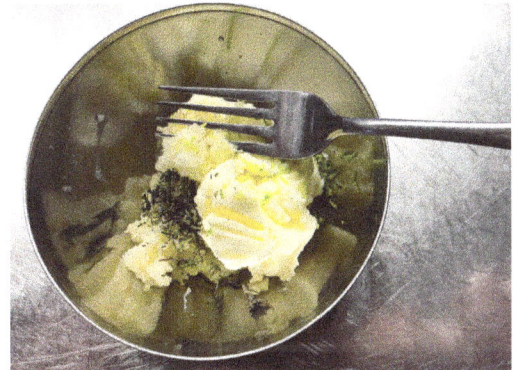

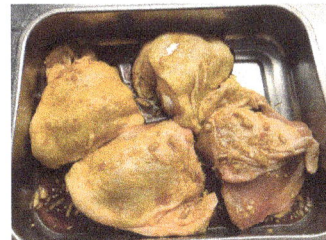

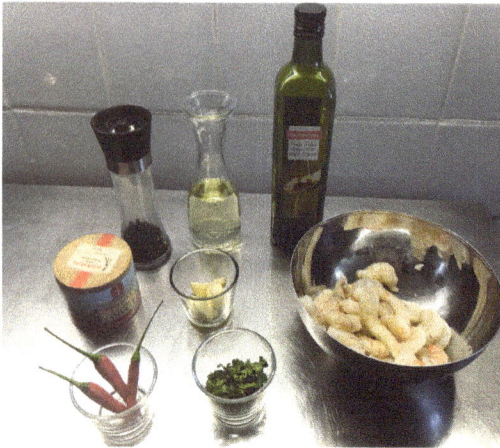

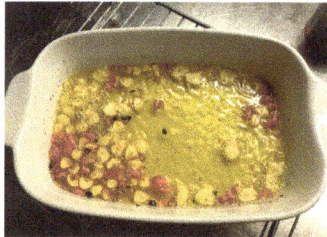

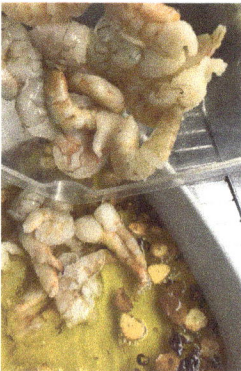

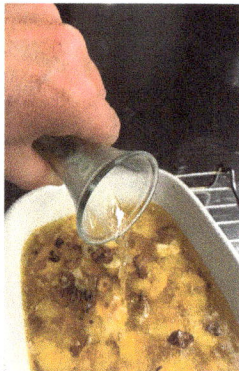

Baked shrimps in spicy oil

24 raw shrimps
150ml olive oil
6 cloves of garlic, sliced
3 peppers, sliced
150ml white wine
Salt, pepper
Chopped parsley

Preheat your oven to 200°C.

Preheat your ceramic oven dish
for about 5 min.

Add the oil, garlic, peppers and salt.
Leave to heat for 3 min.

Add the shrimp and return to the
oven for 6 min.

Deglaze with white wine and
cook for another 2 min.
Season with salt and pepper.
Sprinkle with the parsley.

Serve with fresh crispy bread.

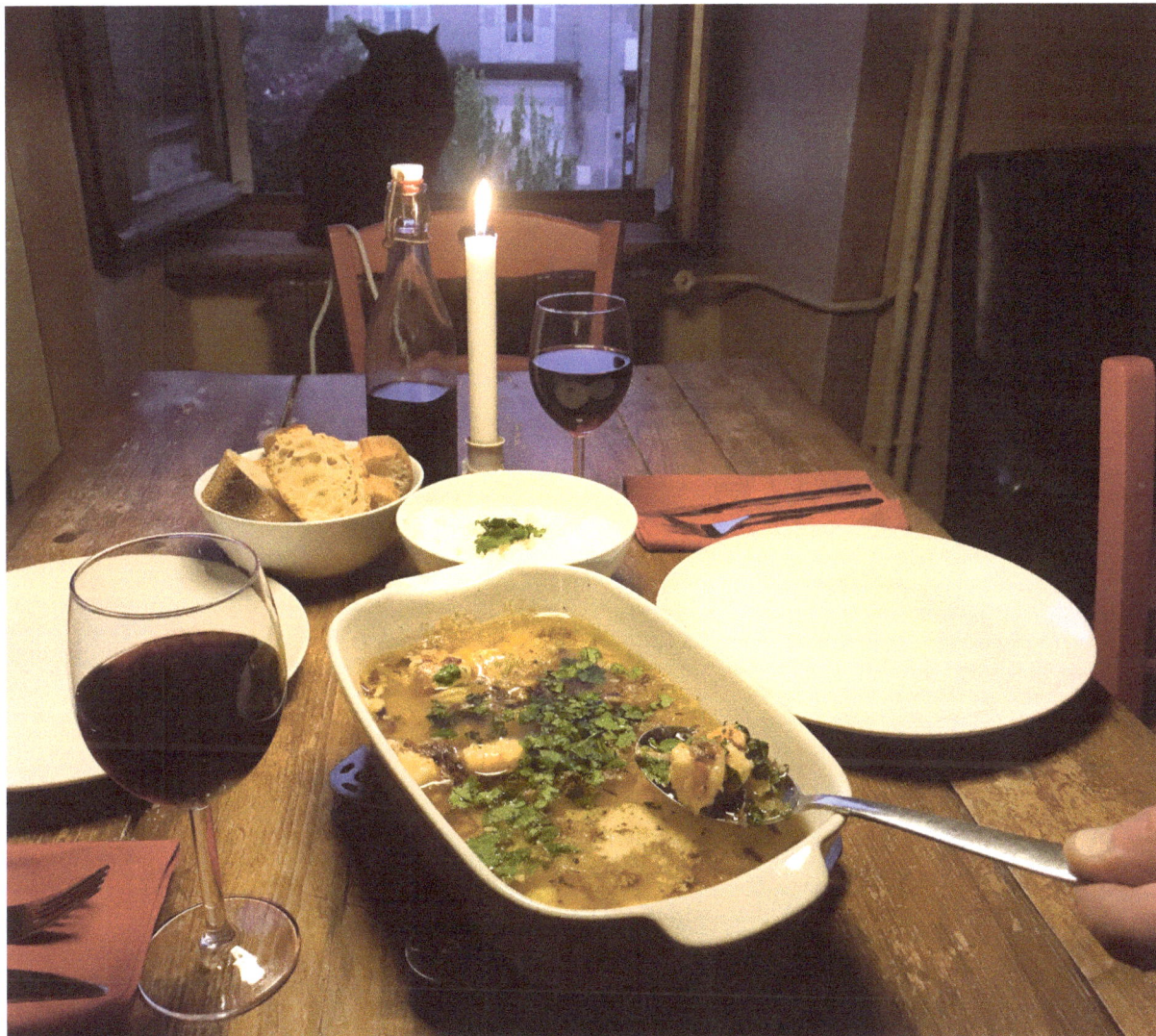

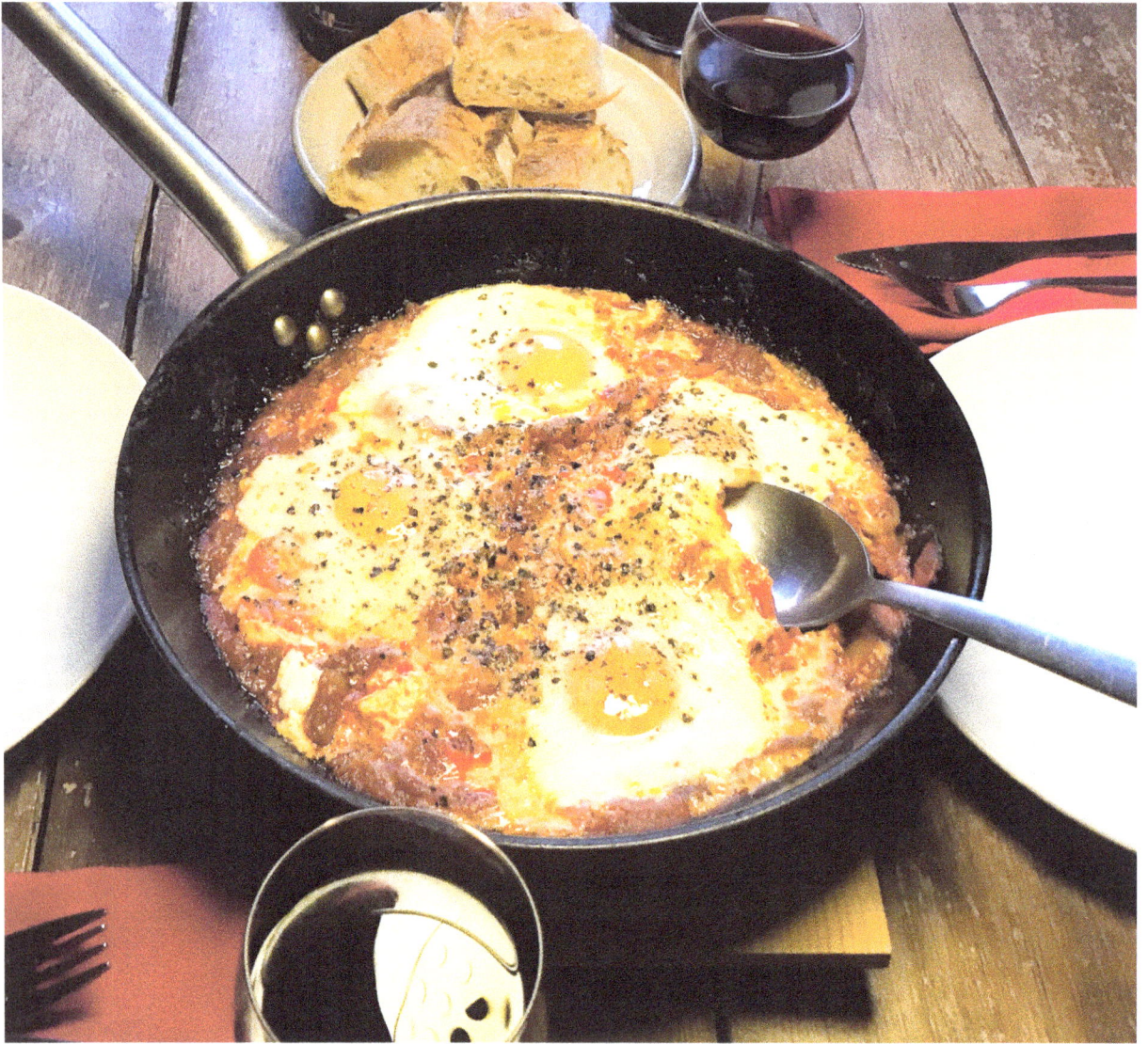

Shakshuka

1 onion, thinly sliced
1/2 red pepper, thinly sliced
2 cloves of garlic, chopped
400g peeled tomatoes
100g diced feta cheese
4 eggs
Olive oil
1/2 tsp sweet ground paprika
1/2 tsp cumin
1/2 tsp ground hot pepper
Coriander or parsley
Salt, pepper

Heat the olive oil in a pan and gently cook
the onions and peppers for about 15 min.

In the last 2 min of cooking, add the garlic.
Add the spices and cook for 30 sec.
Add the tomatoes and mash them.
Simmer for 15 min.

Preheat your oven to 190°C (non-rotating heat).

Add the feta cheese. Season with salt and pepper.

Form 4 small holes in your sauce
and break the eggs into these holes.
Bake for 8–10 min.

Garnish with coriander or parsley.

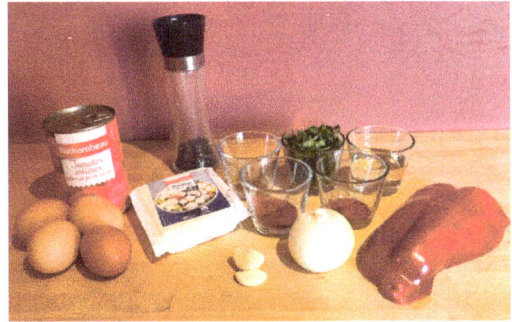

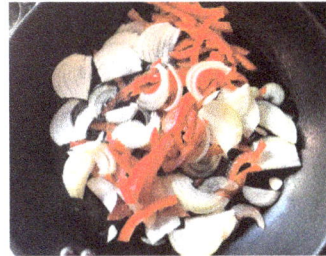

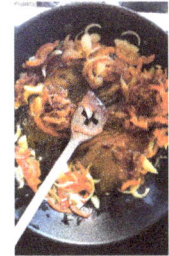

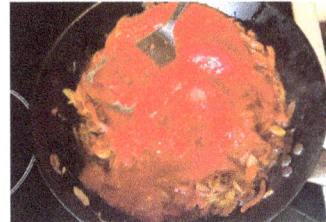

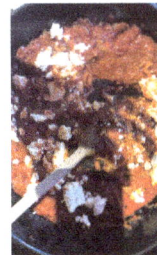

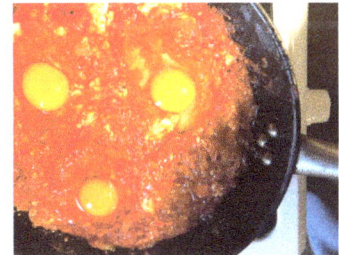

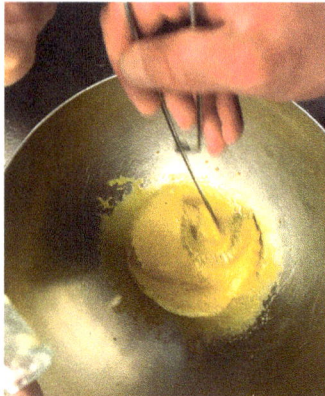

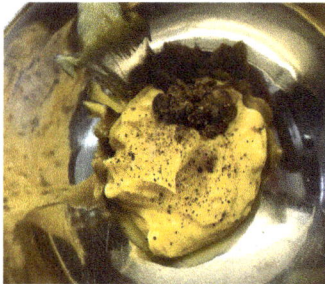

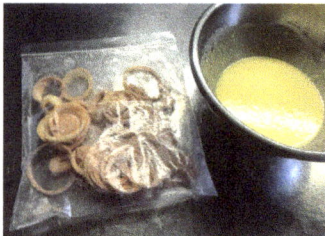

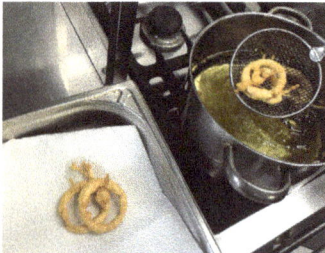

Onion rings and mayonnaise with jalapeños

2 onions, cut into rings
1 egg
120g flour + 30g
30g cornstarch
180ml beer
Sweet paprika powder, salt, pepper
*
1 egg yolk
180ml oil
2 tsp lemon juice
1 tsp mustard
1 tsp Worcestershire sauce
Chopped jalapeños

Prepare a batter with the flour, cornstarch,
egg and beer. Season with salt and pepper.

Put the extra flour and the sweet paprika powder
in a freezer bag. Add the onion rings and shake.

Heat the frying oil in a saucepan to 175°C.

Mix the egg yolk, mustard, lemon juice
and Worcestershire sauce.
Add the oil little by little to prepare your mayonnaise.
Season with the jalapeños and salt.

Dip the onion rings in the batter
and fry them for about 3 min.

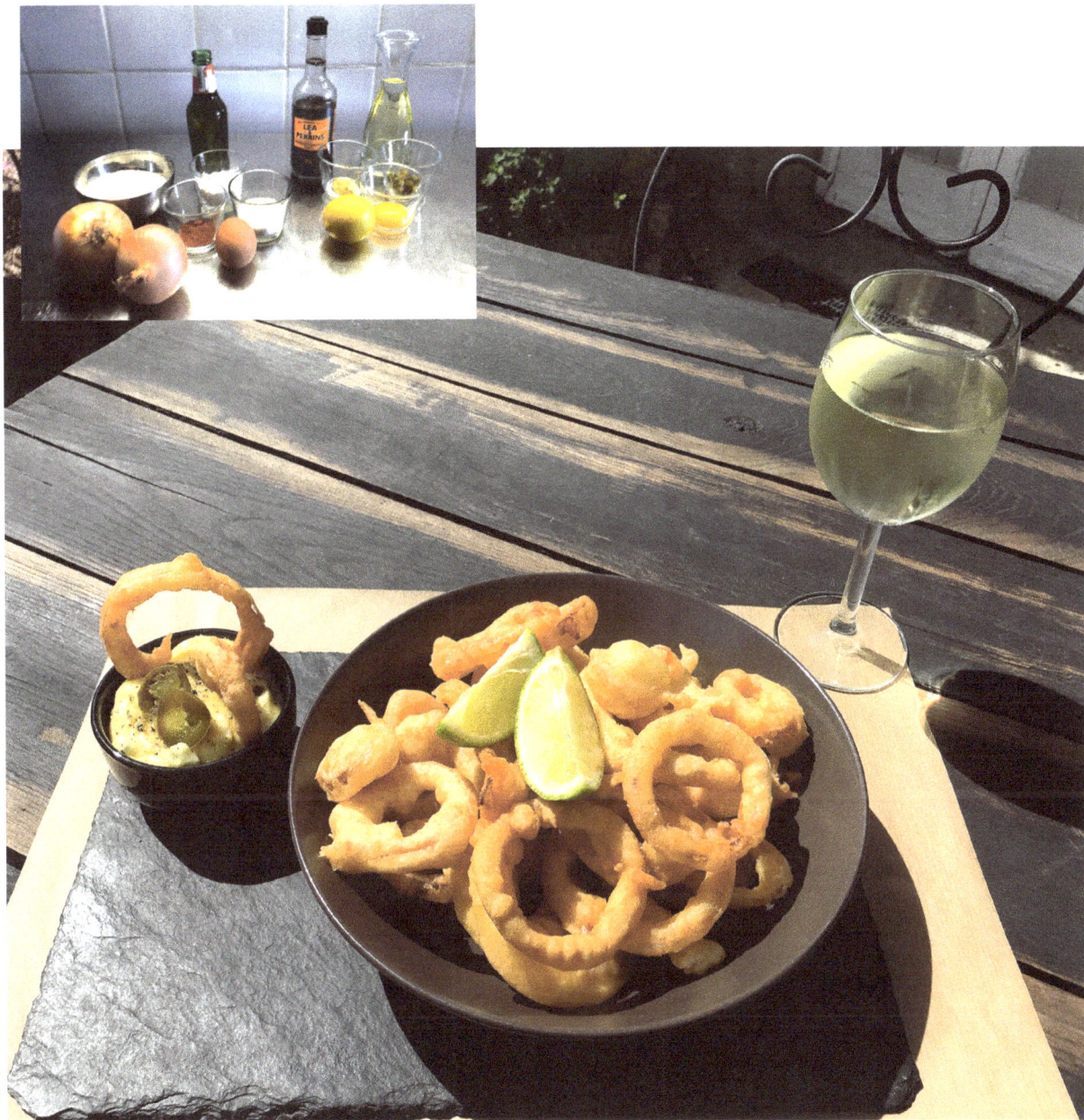

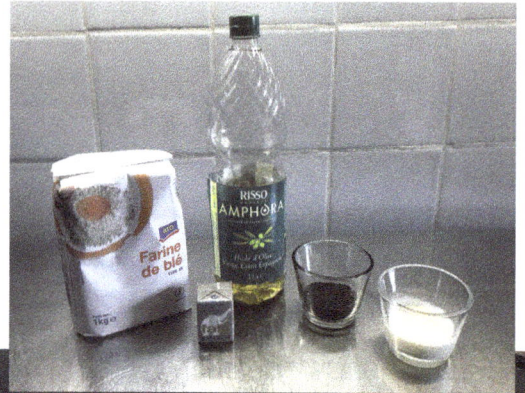

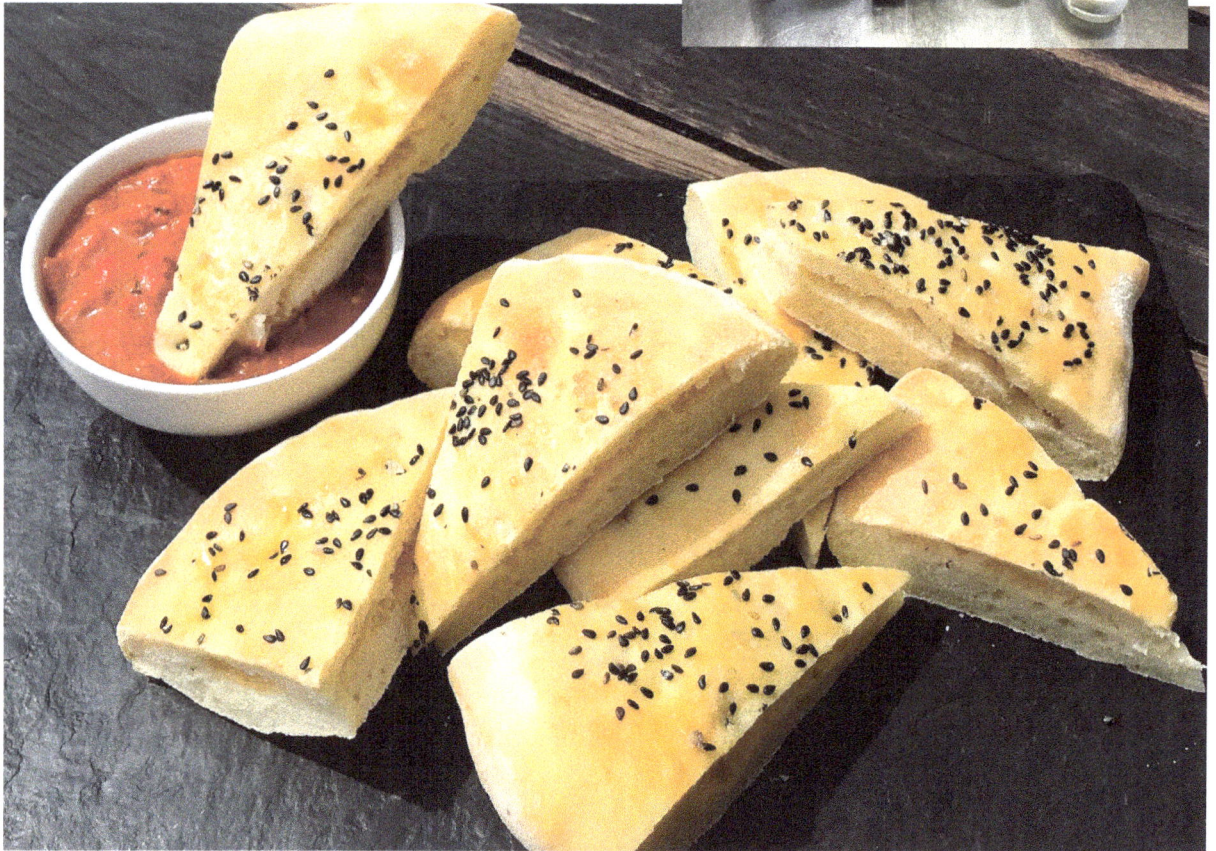

Turkish flatbread

500g flour
1 cube of yeast (or 2 tsp dried yeast)
300ml lukewarm water
1 tsp sugar
Salt
4 tbsp olive oil + 1 tbsp
Milk
Sesame seeds
Fleur de sel

Mix the yeast and sugar in lukewarm water.
Prepare a dough with the flour, baking powder,
olive oil, yeast mixture and a little salt.
Leave it to rise for 1 hr.

Preheat your oven to 210°C.

Divide the dough in half. Roll out the dough
to about 25cm and place on your baking sheet.

Wet your fingers with water and shape
small indentations on the dough.
Brush with milk and sprinkle with sesame seeds
and fleur de sel.

Leave it to rise for 15 min.

Bake for 15–20 min.

Brush with a little olive oil and leave to cool.

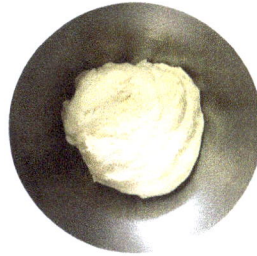

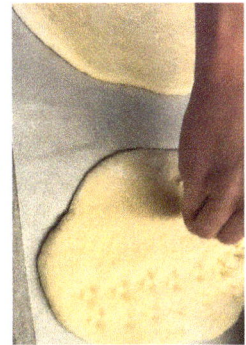

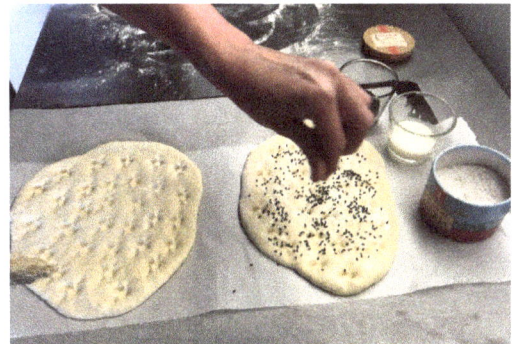

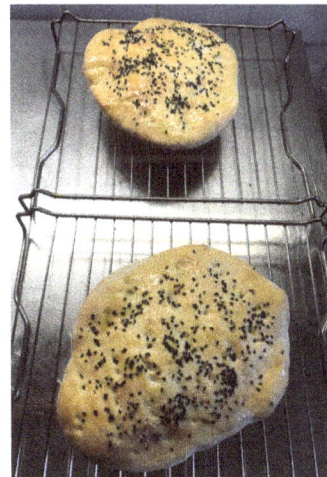

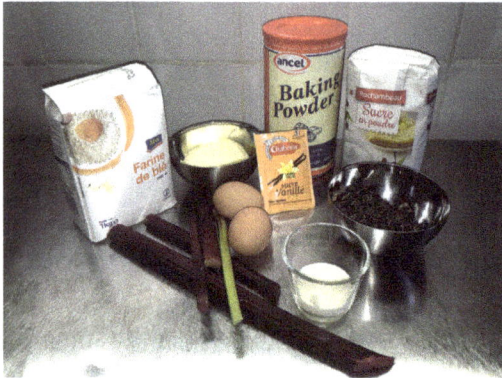

Rhubarb–chocolate cookies

175g soft butter
200g sugar
2 eggs
1 tbsp vanilla sugar
1 tbsp milk
175g chopped chocolate
275g flour
1 tsp baking powder
250g rhubarb, cut into 1cm slices

Preheat your oven to 190°C.

Cream the butter and the sugar with a whisk.
Add the eggs, milk, vanilla sugar and mix
for another 1 min.

Mix in the chocolate, the flour, baking powder
and a pinch of salt. Add to the mixture of butter, eggs
and sugar. Gently fold in the rhubarb slices.

Place the dough in 1 tbsp scoops on
your baking tray.

Cook for 10 min.

Remove from the oven.

Lower the temperature of your oven to 100°C.
Bake your cookies and let them 'dry'
for another 20 min.

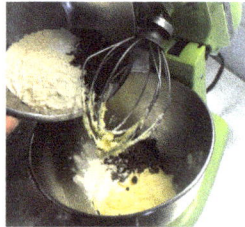

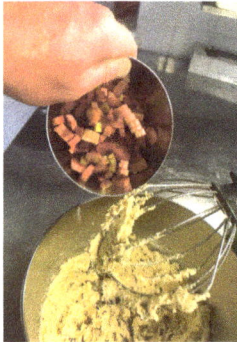

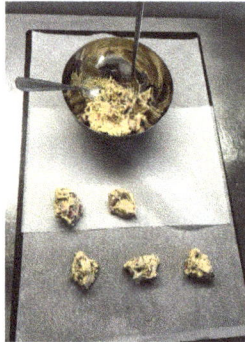

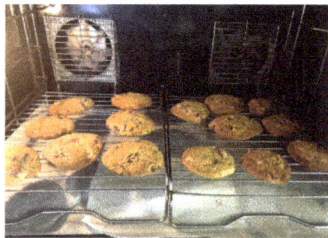

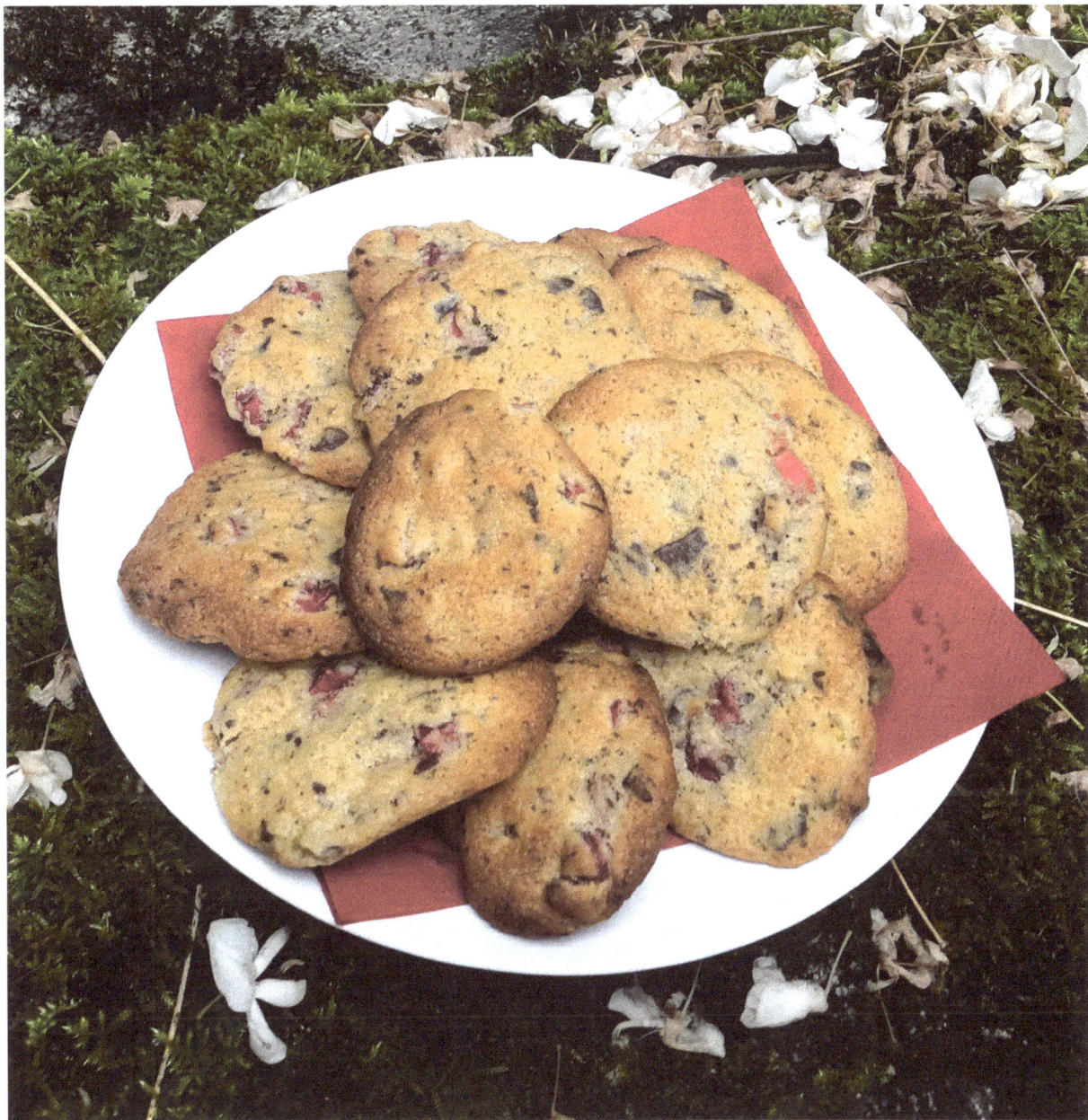

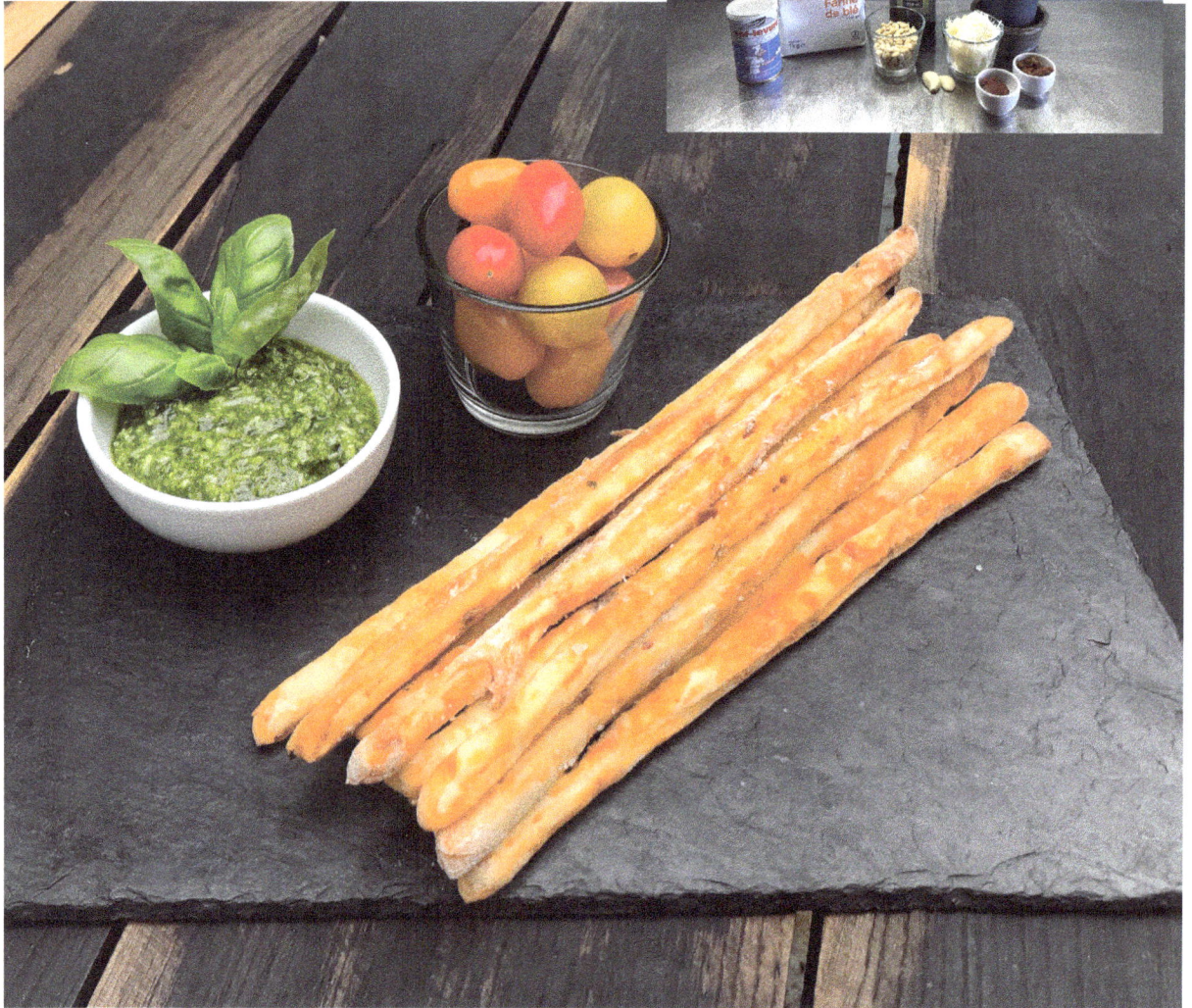

Tomato grissini with basil pesto

125g flour
50ml lukewarm water
3–4g dry yeast
3 tbsp olive oil + a little extra (or chilli oil)
1/2 tbsp tomato paste
2 sun-dried tomatoes, chopped
Salt
*
50g basil leaves
40g grated Parmesan cheese
30g roasted pine nuts
2 cloves of garlic
110ml olive oil
Fleur de sel

Leave the yeast to act in lukewarm water.
Prepare a dough with the flour, yeast mixture, olive oil
and a little salt. Add the tomato paste and the sundried
tomatoes. Leave it to rest for 45–60 min.

Preheat your oven to 190°C.

For the pesto, mix the basil leaves, olive oil, garlic
and pine nuts and blend it until you achieve a
smooth consistency. Add the Parmesan and mix well
with a fork (do not blend).

Roll out the dough to about 1cm thickness and
cut into strips. Roll the strips and place them
on your baking sheet. Brush with olive oil and
sprinkle with fleur de sel. Bake for 12 min.
Allow to cool.

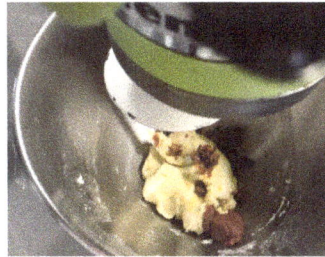
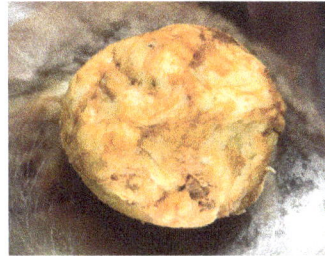
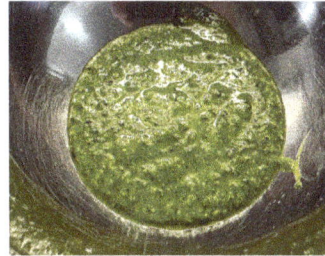
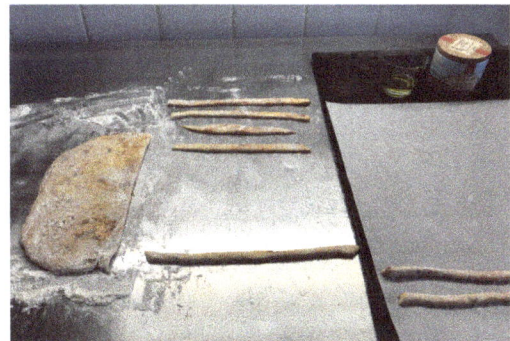

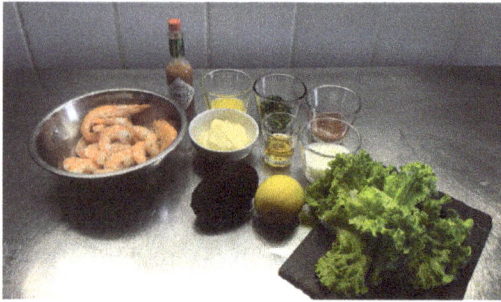

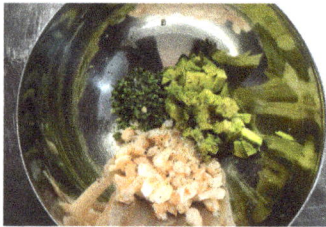

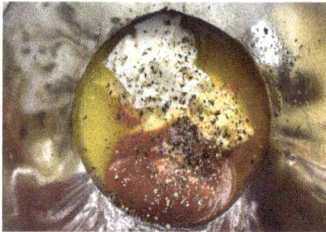

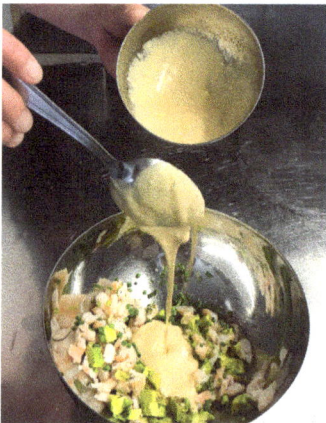

Shrimp and avocado cocktail

300g pre-cooked shrimps
1 avocado
1 1/2 tbsp mayonnaise
(Recipe of Day 24, without jalapeños)
1 tbsp yogurt
1/2 tbsp ketchup
1/4 tsp cognac (optional)
1/2 tsp orange juice
Juice of one lemon
Tabasco sauce
Chopped chives
A few salad leaves cut into thin strips
Salt, pepper

Half the avocado, remove the flesh with
a spoon and cut into cubes.
Chop the shrimp into small slices.

For the sauce, mix the mayonnaise, ketchup,
yogurt, brandy and orange juice. Season with
Tabasco sauce, lemon juice, salt and pepper.

Mix the shrimp pieces and avocado cubes
with the sauce and chives.

Add the salad leaves and mix well.

Fill the empty avocado skins
with the cocktail mixture.

Garnish with lemon slices, salad
and additional shrimps.

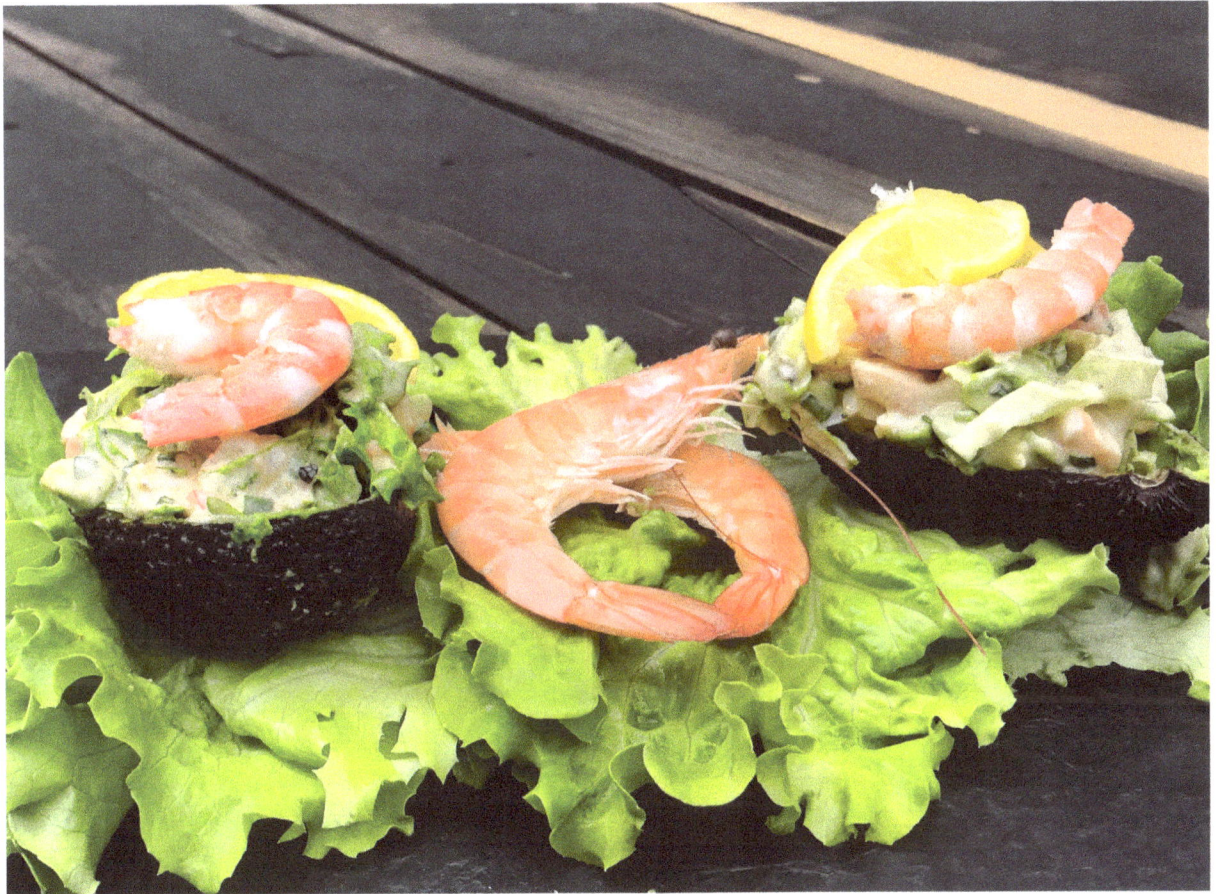

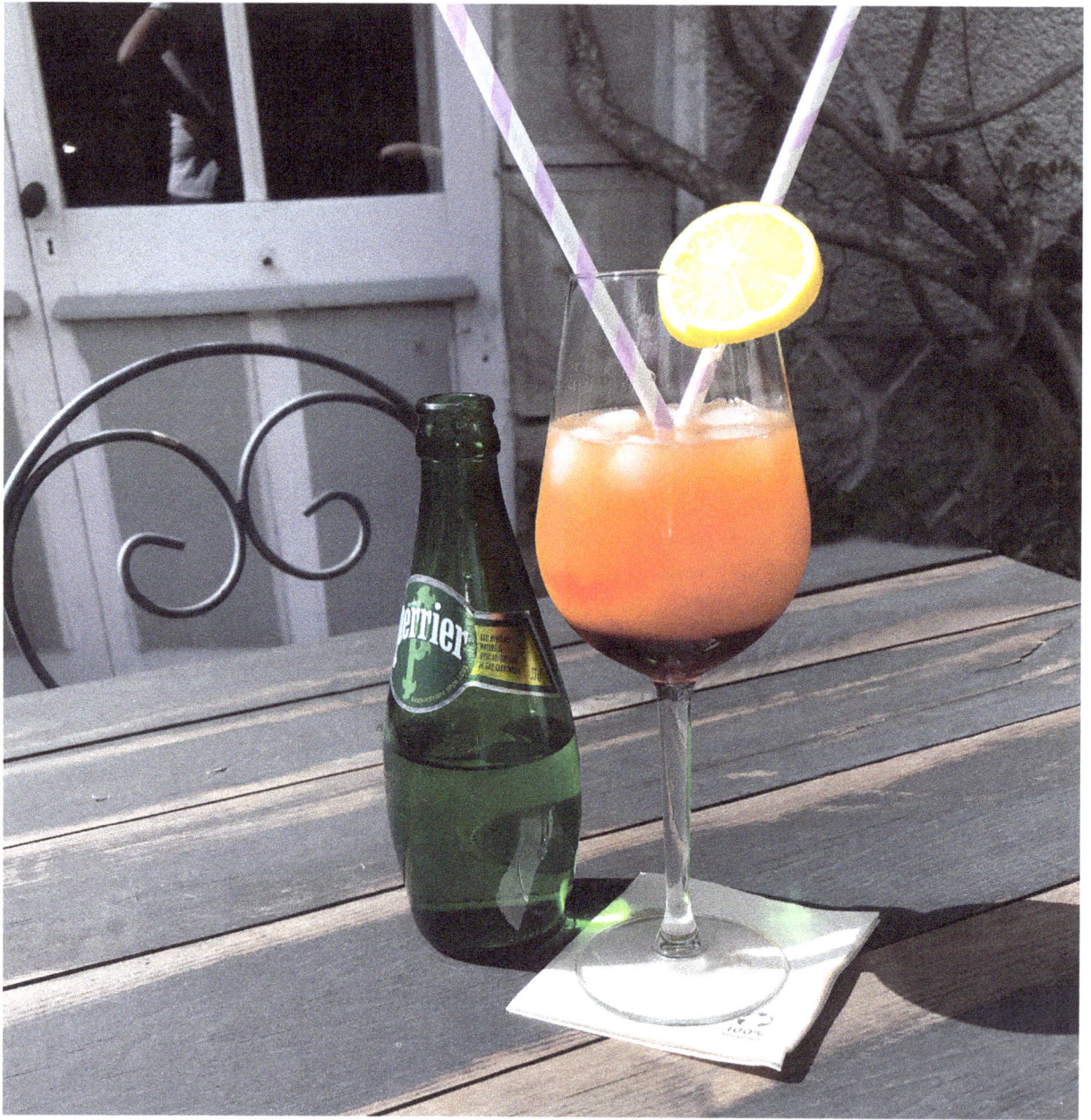

Le Sens de la Terre house aperitif

(non-alcoholic*)

12cl mango juice
4cl Grenadine syrup
Sparkling water
1 hibiscus flower
1–2 lemon slices
Angostura Bitters (optional, with alcohol*)
Ice cubes

Pour a few drops of Angostura Bitters in a glass.

Add the Grenadine syrup and ice cubes.

Slowly add mango juice, pouring
it over a teaspoon.

Place the hibiscus flower in the middle
of the glass.

Fill the glass with the sparkling water.

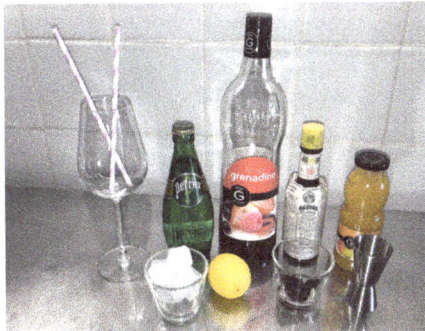

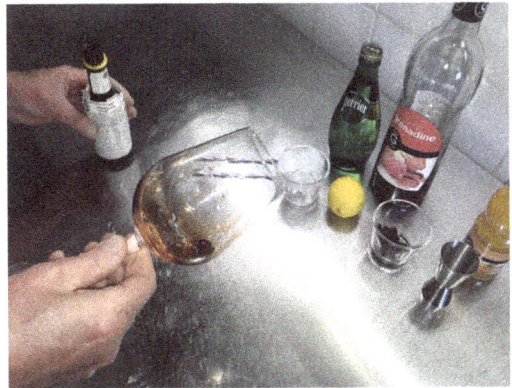

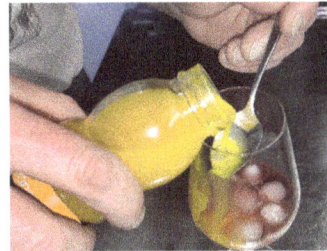

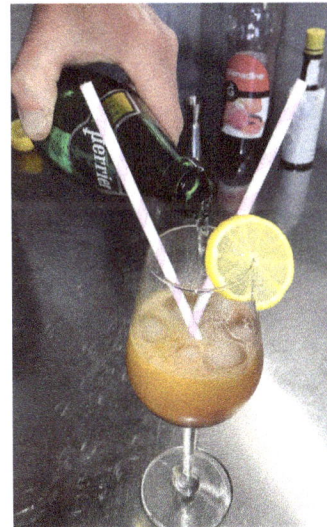

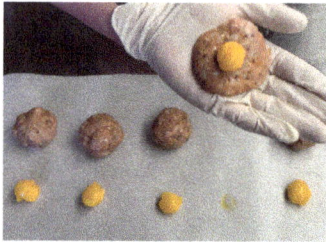

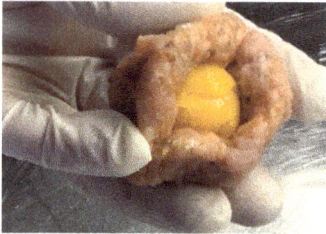

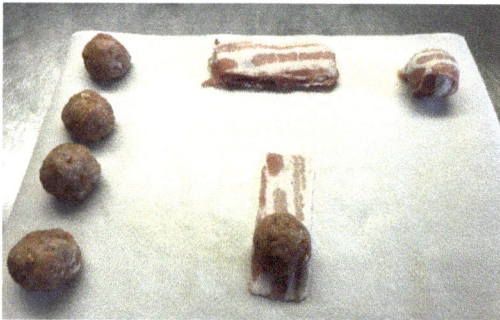

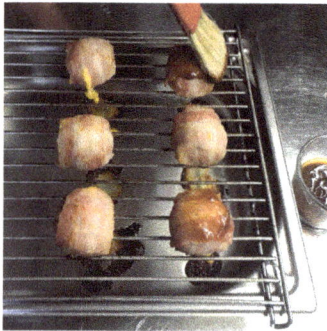

Mini bacon bombs
(makes 6)

180g minced meat
40g melted cheddar cheese
6 slices bacon
1/2 red onion chopped into small cubes ('brunoise')
1 garlic clove, minced
1/2 tsp ground paprika
1/2 tsp dried oregano
1/2 tsp mustard
Tabasco sauce
Salt, pepper
2–3 tbsp BBQ sauce *(see recipe for Day 12)*

Mix the minced meat with the garlic, onion,
mustard and herbs. Add a few drops of Tabasco sauce
and season with salt and pepper.

Preheat your oven to 180°C (or your BBQ).

Form small balls of approximately 30g of minced meat
as well as small balls of melted cheddar. Flatten the
meatballs and place a cheddar ball in the centre.
Reform the meatballs.

Cut the bacon in half lengthwise and encircle
a meatball with one of the bacon strips. Repeat with
the other bacon strip so it encircles the meatball at
right angles to the first strip. Repeat the operation
on each meatball.

Place your meatballs on your baking sheet
and cook for 20 min.

Remove from the oven and brush your meatballs
with BBQ sauce.

Return to the oven (220°C, grill function)
for 5–7 min.

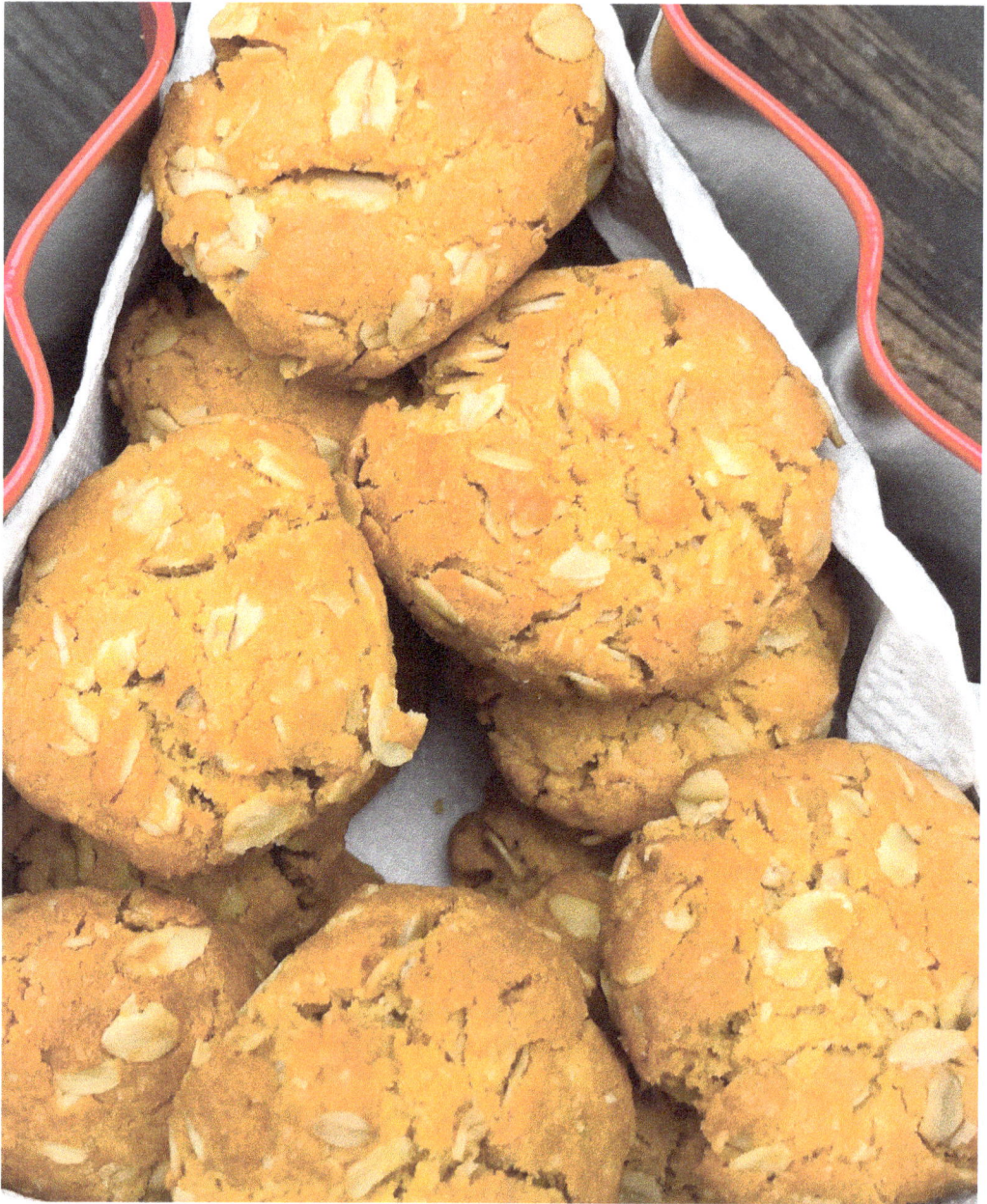

ANZAC cookies

125g butter
150g flour
l00g honey
100g oatmeal
75g grated coconut flakes
1/2 tsp baking soda
2 tsp water
Salt

Preheat your oven to 150°C.

Melt the butter and add the honey.

Dissolve the baking soda in the water, then add it, with a pinch of salt, to the butter and honey mixture.

Mix all the dry ingredients and add them to the butter mixture to form a paste.

Form small balls (about 1 tsp) and place them on your baking sheet.

Bake for 20 min.

Allow to cool.

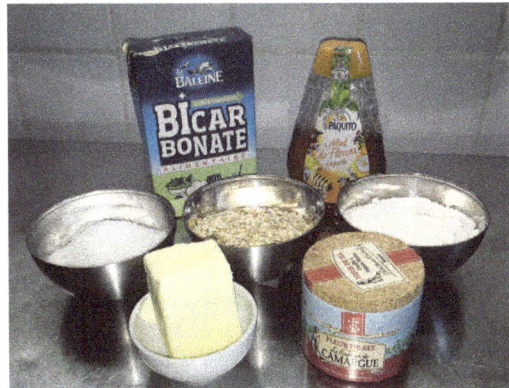

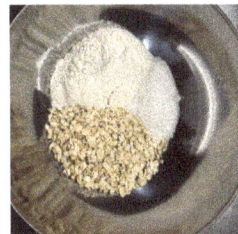
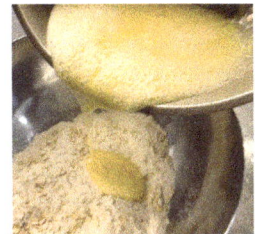

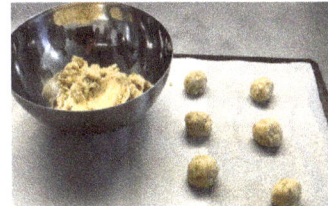

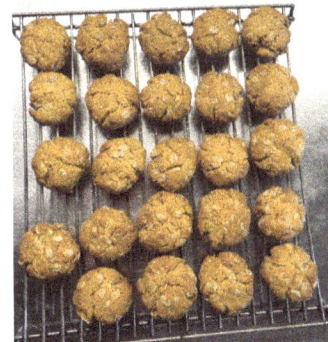

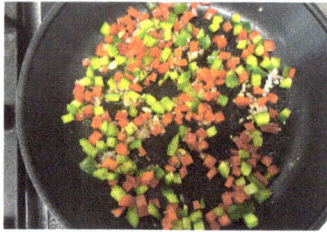

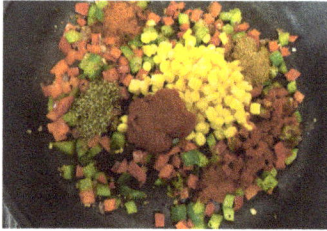

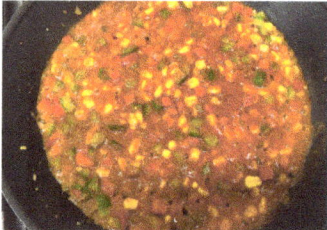

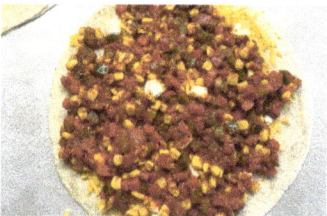

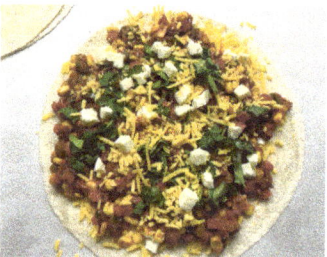

Quesadillas (v)

2 wheat tortillas
1/2 red bell pepper, 1/2 green bell pepper, diced
70g sweet corn
1/2 red onion, finely chopped ('brunoise')
1 clove of garlic
1/2 tbsp tomato paste
60ml water
50g grated cheddar cheese
50g diced mozzarella
1 tsp oregano, 1 tsp sweet paprika,
1 tsp cumin, 1/4 tsp hot pepper powder
Coriander
Salt, pepper

Heat a little olive oil in a pan and brown the onion
and chopped garlic for 1–2 min. Add the diced peppers
and fry for 2 min. Add the tomato paste, herbs,
sweet corn and water. Leave to cook for 3–4 min.

Season with salt and pepper and let cool.

Take a tortilla and place half the cheeses on it.
Cover with sauce and sprinkle a little coriander.

Add the other half of the cheeses and place
the second tortilla on top.

Heat a pan and fry your quesadilla
for about 4 min on low heat.

Flip and cook the other side
for another 3–4 min.

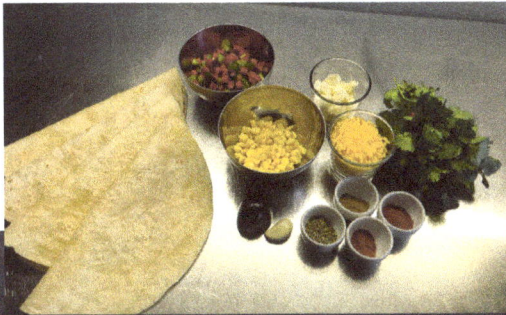

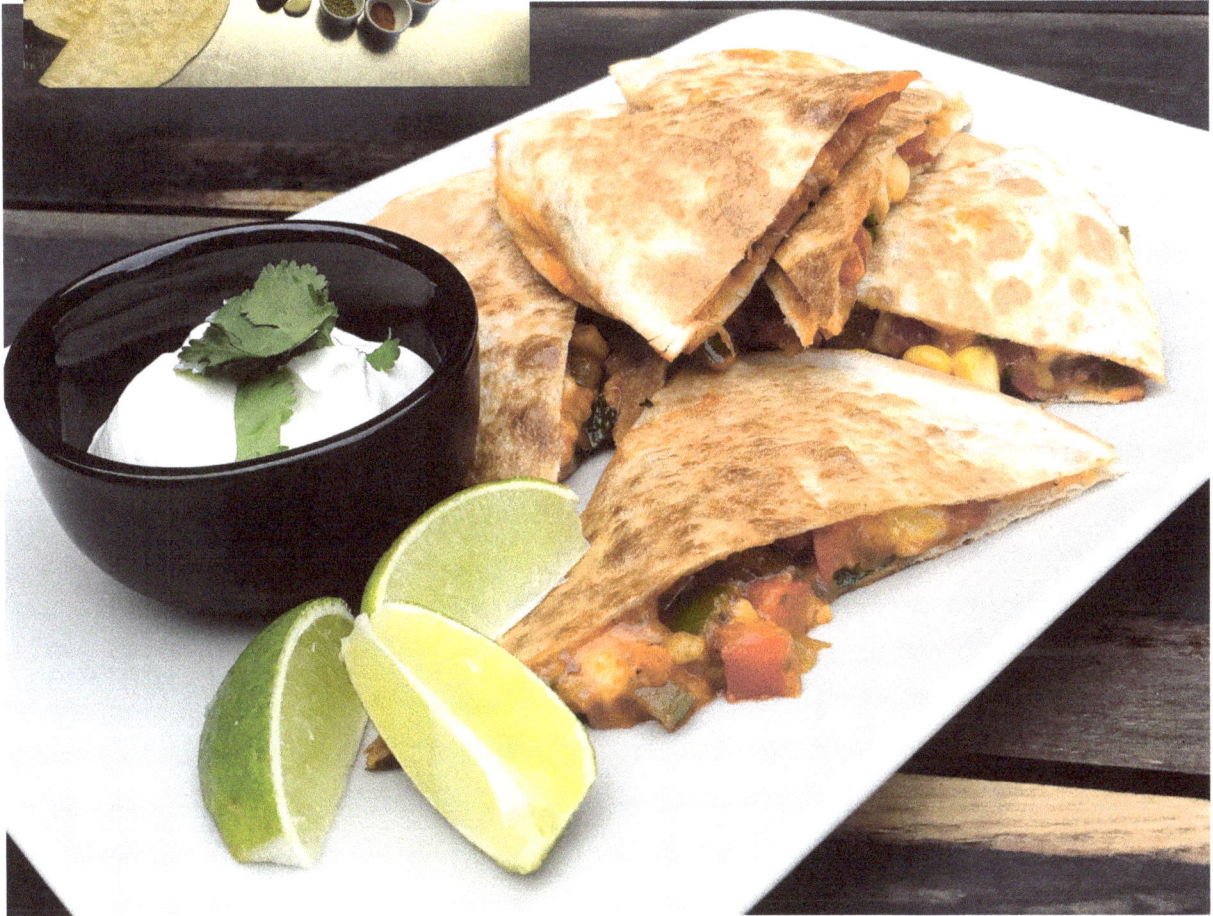

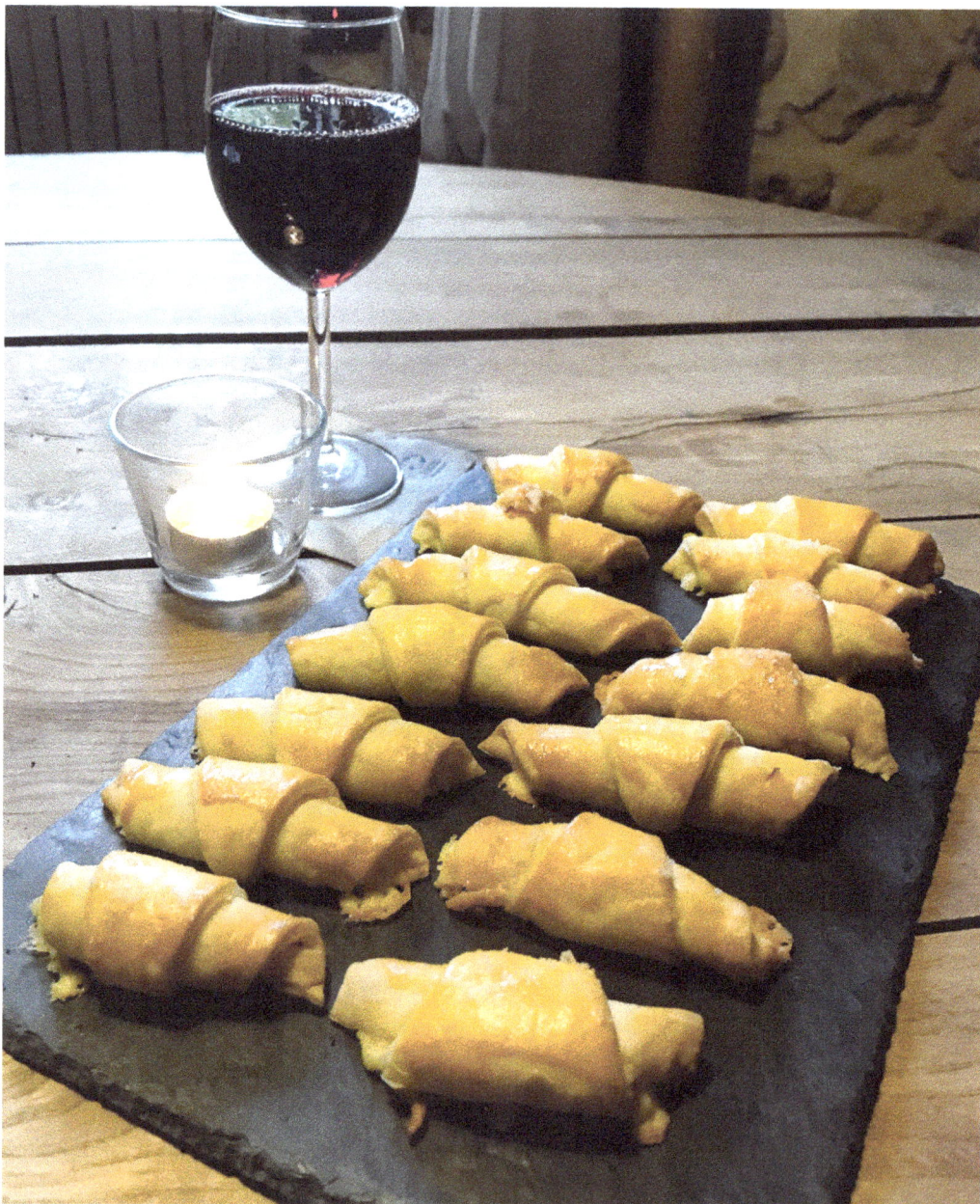

Mini ham and cheese croissants

150g flour
100g soft butter
100g cream cheese (Philadelphia)
1/2 tsp salt
4 slices of ham
100g grated Gouda cheese
1 egg
Fleur de sel

Prepare a smooth dough with the flour, butter,
cream cheese and a pinch of salt.

Form a ball and let it rest in the fridge for 2 hr.

Cut the ham into 16 triangles.

Preheat your oven to 175°C.

Divide the dough in half and roll it out
into a rectangle about 25cm long.

Cut each half into 8 triangles of dough.

Place your ham and cheese on it.
Roll the dough into small 'croissants'.

Brush with beaten egg and sprinkle
with fleur de sel.

Bake for 15–20 min.

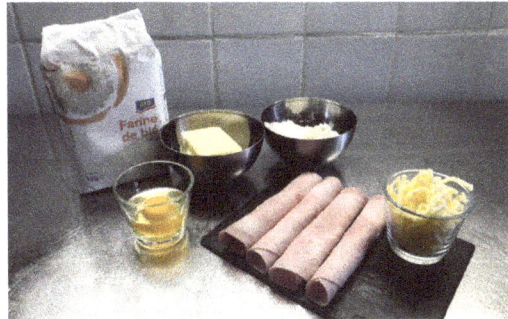

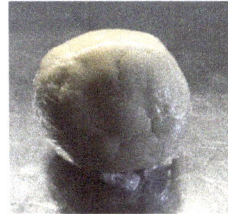

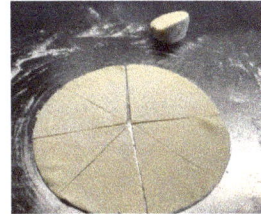

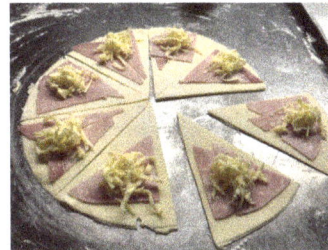

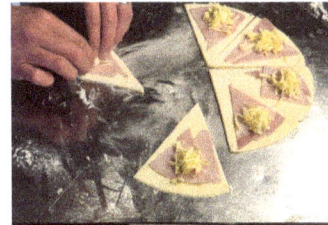

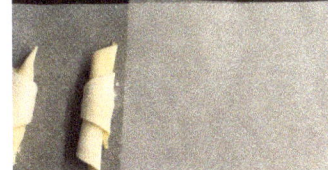

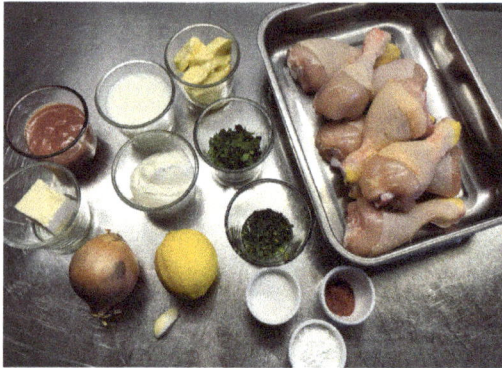

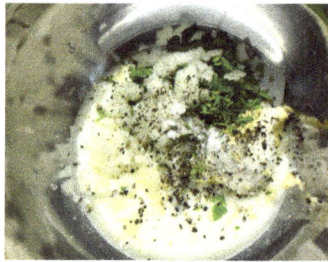

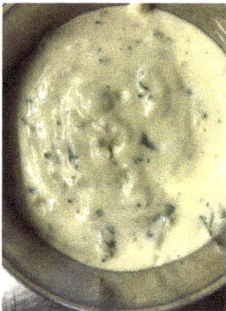

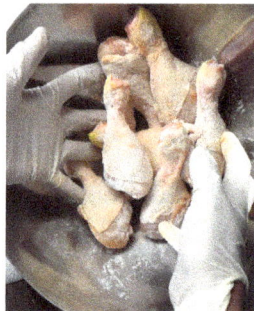

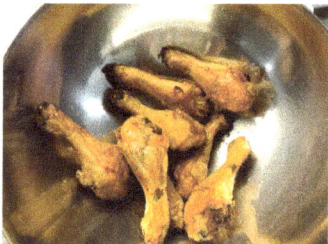

'Buffalo' chicken drumsticks

8 chicken drumsticks
2 1/2 tsp baking powder
1 tsp ground sweet paprika
30g melted butter
70ml sriracha sauce
1/2 tsp sugar
Salt, pepper

*

75g mayonnaise, 75g yogurt
75ml buttermilk
1/2 chopped onion, 1/2 garlic clove, chopped
1/2 tsp chopped parsley, 1/2 tsp chopped chives
1/2 tsp lemon juice

Preheat your oven to 120°C.

Dry the chicken drumsticks and mix with the baking
powder, sweet paprika and salt. Place them on
a baking sheet and cook for 30 min.

Mix the mayonnaise, yogurt and buttermilk
with onion, garlic, herbs, lemon juice and
season with salt and pepper.

After 30 min, raise the temperature of your oven
to 220°C and roast the chicken drumsticks
for another 40 min.

Heat the sriracha sauce with the butter.

When your chicken drumsticks are ready, put them
in a bowl and pour on the srichia/butter sauce.

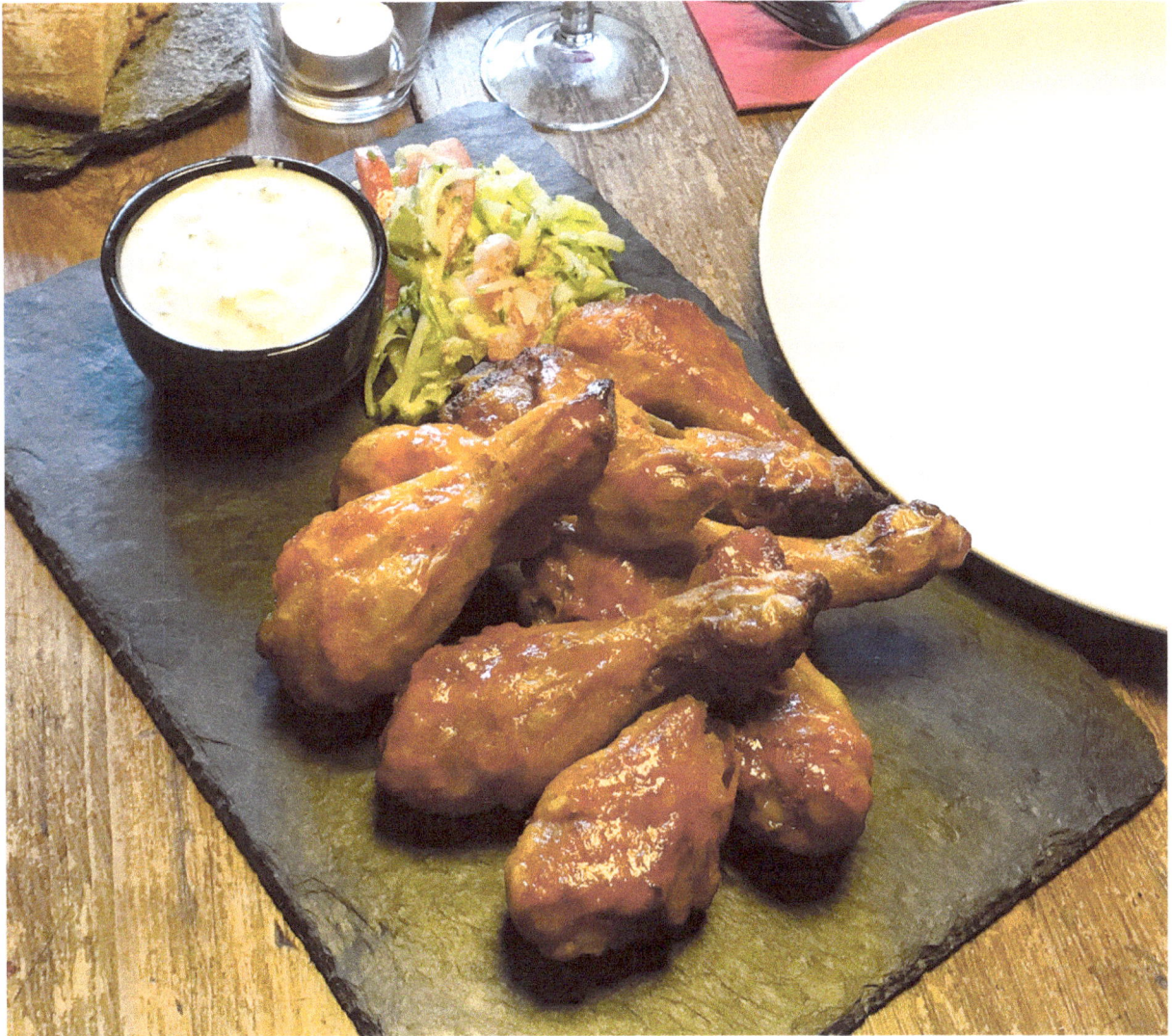

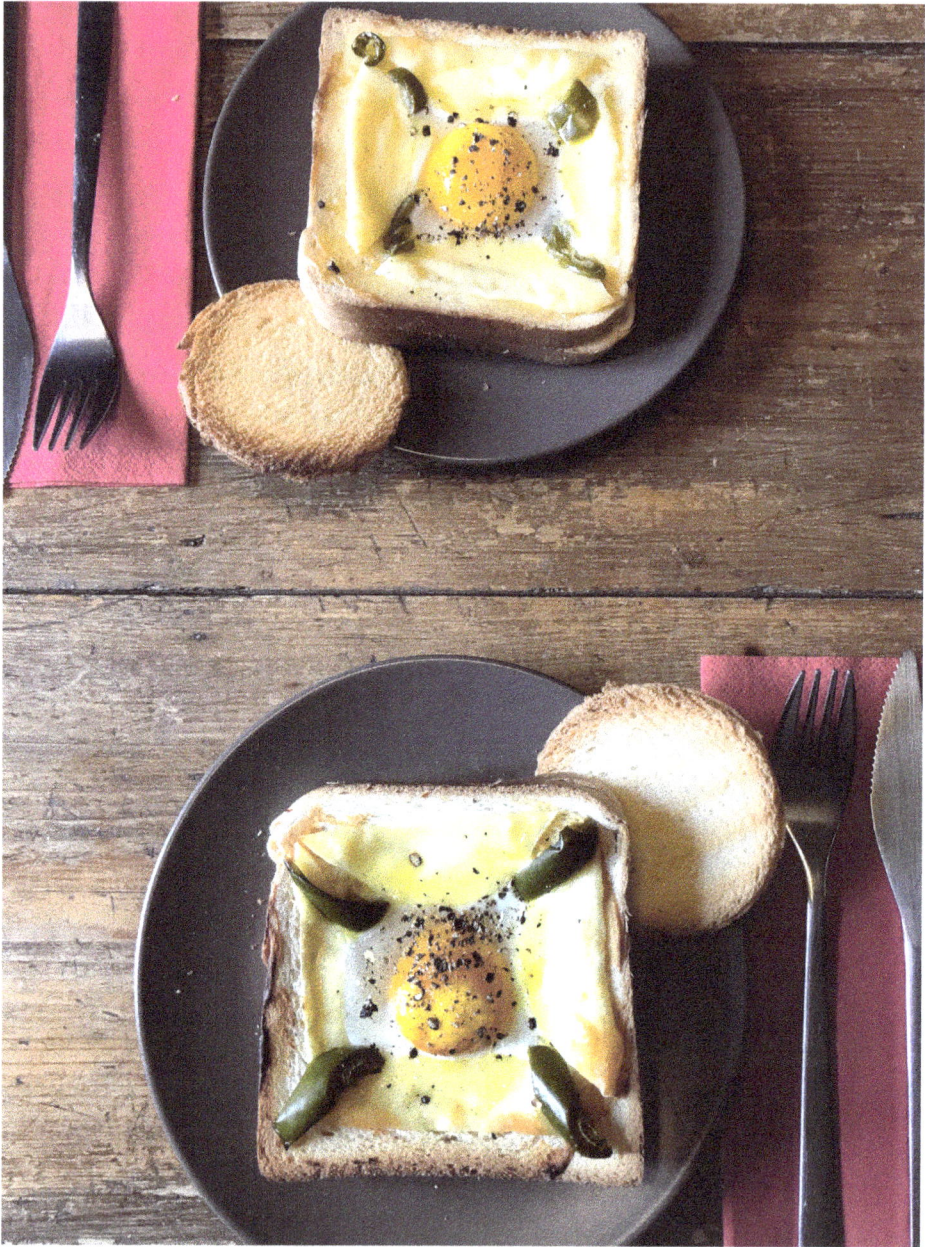

Hole in a toad

4 slices of sandwich bread
2 eggs
2 slices of ham
2 slices of cheese (cut into 8 pieces)
1 tbsp mayonnaise
1 tsp jalapeño mustard (optional)
Pepper

Preheat your oven to 180°C.

Spread two slices of sandwich bread
with mustard. Place the ham and mayonnaise
on the bread.

In the other 2 slices of sandwich bread,
cut out a circle in the middle using a cup.
Place on the toast with the ham.

Break an egg into each hole
and arrange the cheese around.

Season with pepper.

Cook on a baking sheet for 10–15 min.

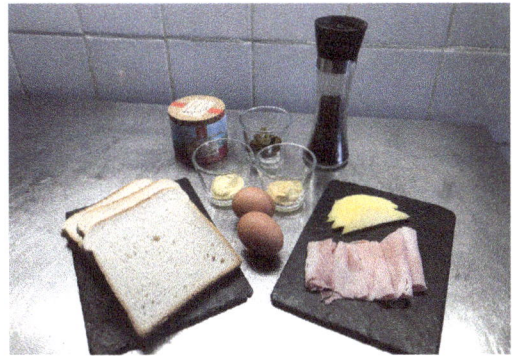

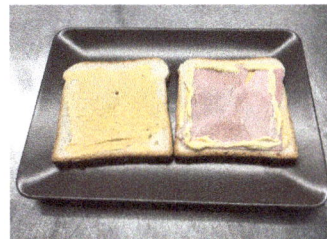

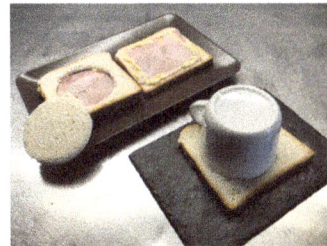

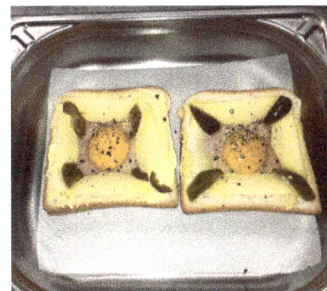

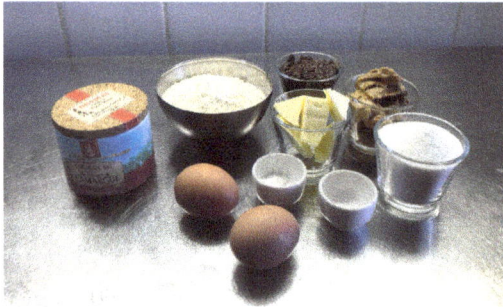

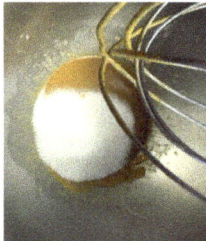

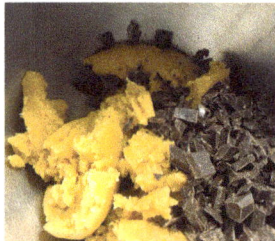

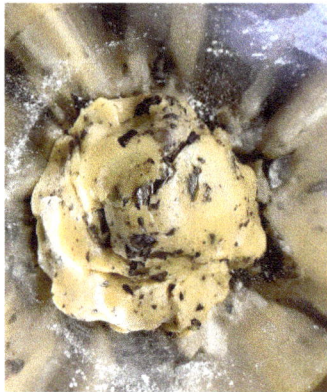

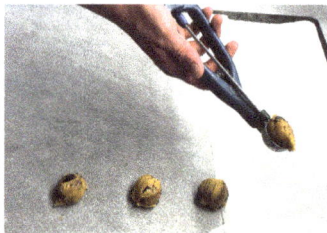

Chocolate peanut butter cookies

160g flour
120g sugar
100g peanut butter
55g melted butter
1 egg + 1 egg yolk
100g chopped dark chocolate
1/2 tsp baking powder
1/2 tsp baking soda
1/2 tsp fleur de sel

Mix the flour with the baking powder,
baking soda and fleur de sel.

Mix the melted butter with the peanut butter,
add the sugar and mix well.

Gradually add the egg and egg yolk.

Add the dry ingredients.
Drop in the chopped chocolate and mix
to a paste. Cover with cling film and
let stand in the fridge for 15–20 min.

Preheat your oven to 175°C.

With the help of an ice cream scoop, place
small balls of dough on a baking sheet.
Lightly crush the balls with your hand.

Bake for 15–20 min.
Let cool.

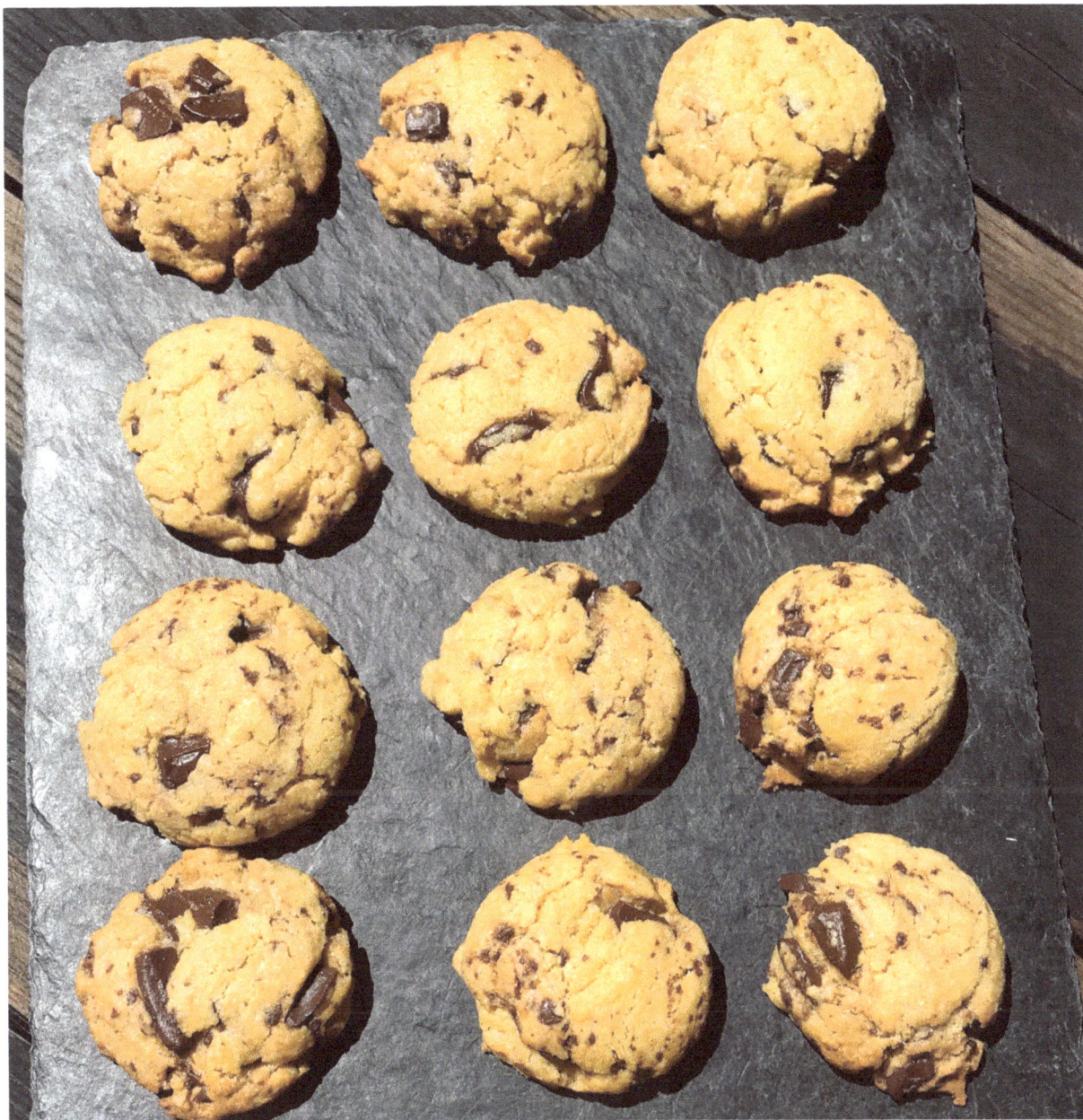

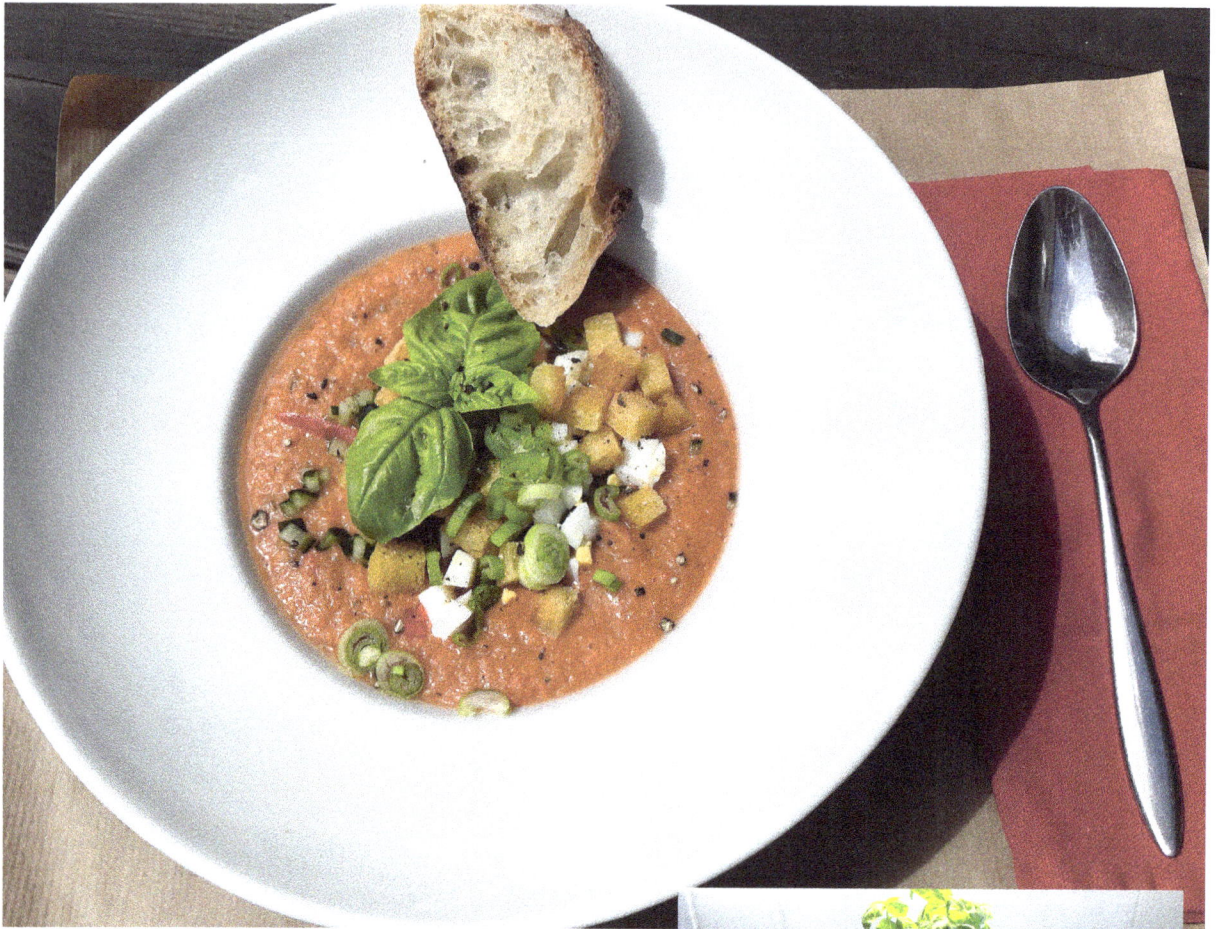

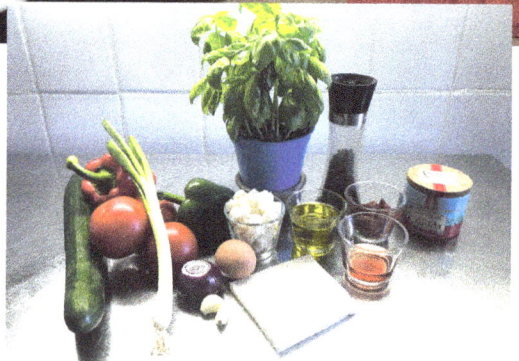

Gazpacho
(serves 2–4)

3 large tomatoes
1/2 red pepper, 1/2 green pepper
1 red onion
2 cloves of garlic
1/4 cucumber
2 tbsp tomato paste
1 slice of white bread
4 tbsp red vinegar
50ml olive oil
Salt, pepper

For garnish:
Red pepper in small cubes
Cucumber, finely chopped ('brunoise')
1 egg, hard-boiled
Chopped spring onions
1 slice of white bread

Cut a slice of sandwich bread into cubes.
Heat a little olive oil in a pan and fry the
bread pieces into croutons.

Dice your vegetables and mix them with the oil olive,
sandwich bread, vinegar, tomato paste, salt and pepper.

Blend to the desired consistency. Season with salt,
pepper, a little more vinegar and olive oil.

Serve with diced peppers and cucumber, chopped
egg, spring onion and croutons.

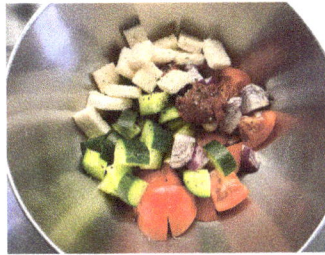

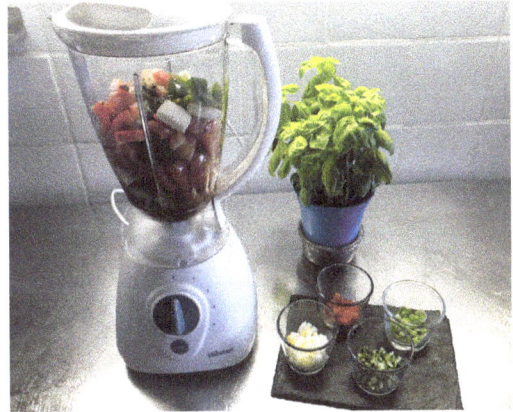

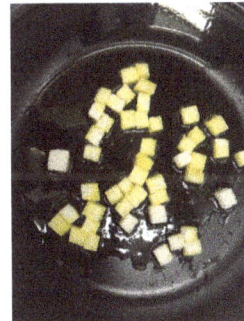

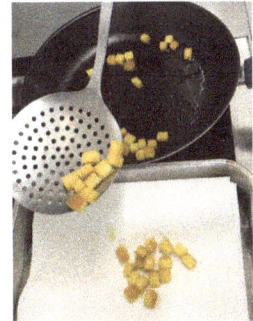

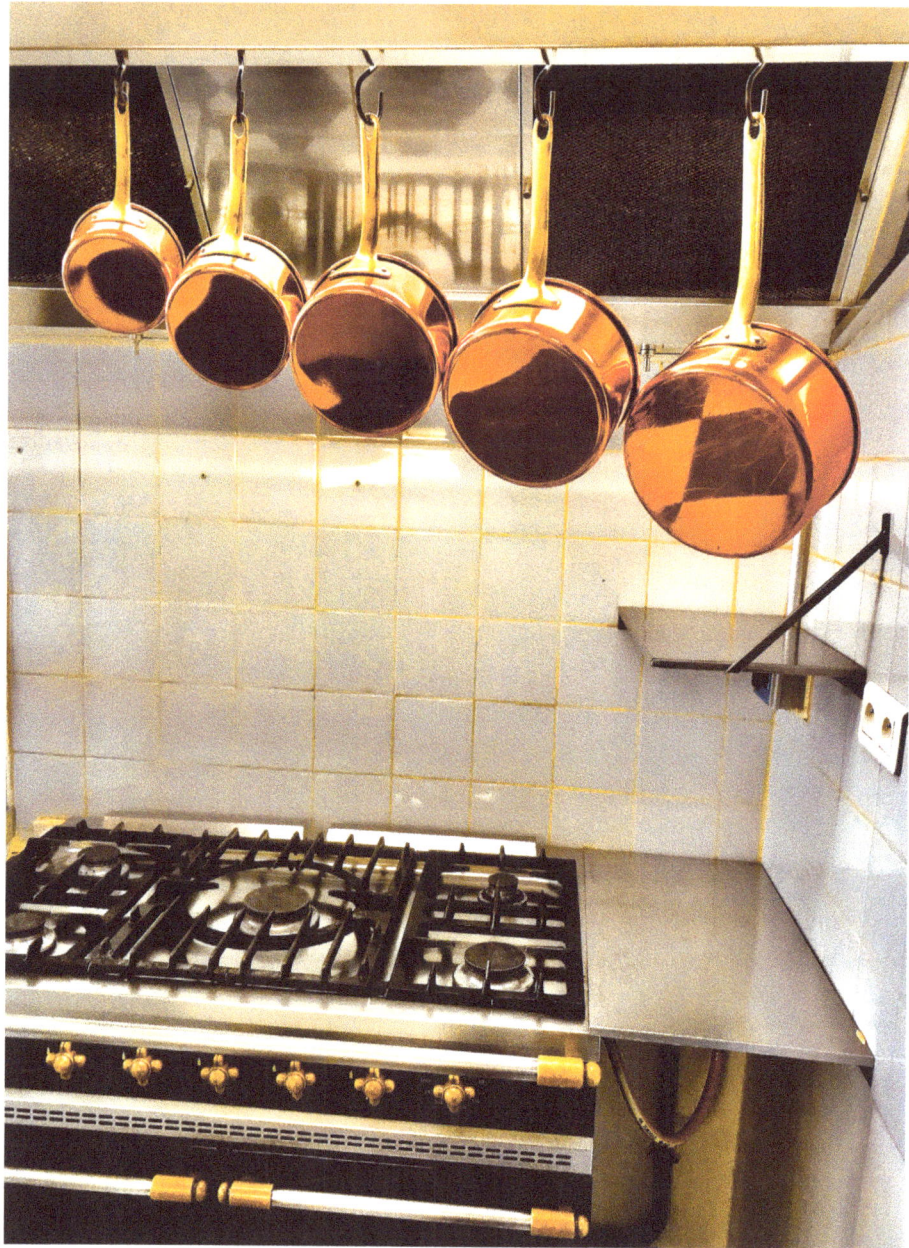

Week 6 of self-isolation

Leo, I'm fed up, I AM <u>NOT</u> GOING TO COOK TODAY...

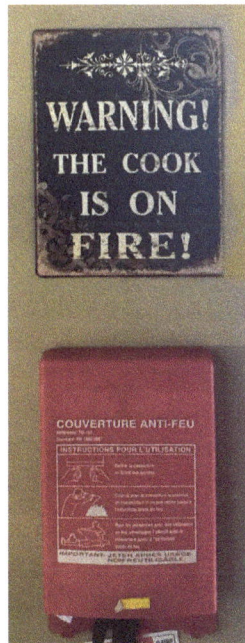

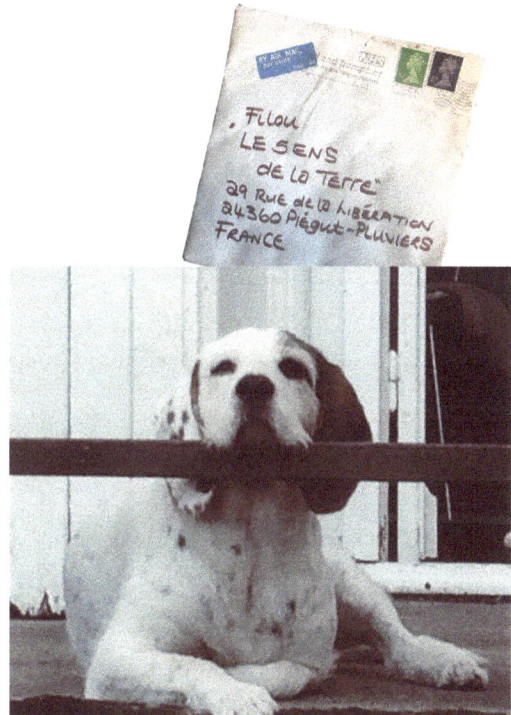

*Nothing to eat tonight? I think I'll go
and live somewhere else..*

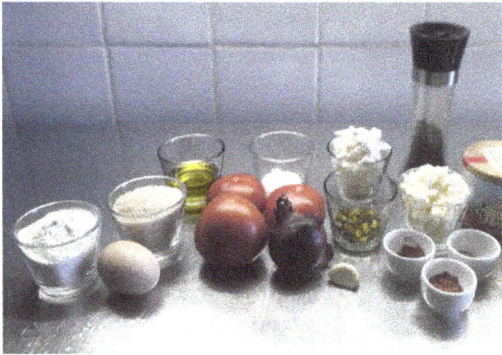

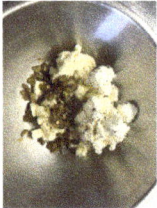

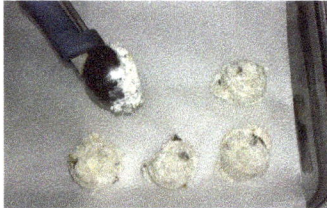

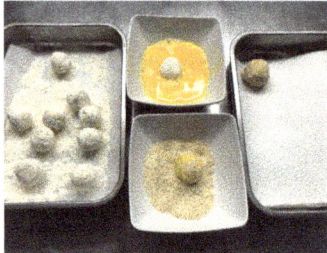

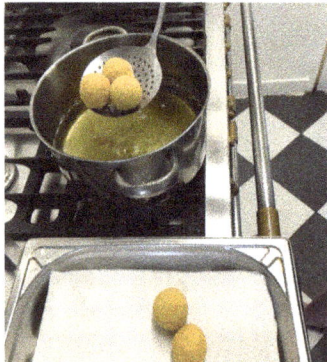

Cheese and jalapeño croquettes

120g diced mozzarella cheese
100g cream cheese
4–6 slices chopped jalapeños
20g breadcrumbs

*

3 tomatoes
1 red onion, diced
1 close of garlic, minced
20ml olive oil
20ml red vinegar
1/2 tsp ground sweet paprika
1/2 tsp ground hot pepper
1/2 tsp cumin, 1 tbsp sugar

*

Breadcrumbs, flour, egg

Mix the mozzarella, cream cheese, breadcrumbs
and jalapeños. Season with salt and pepper.
Form 12 small balls with an ice cream scoop
and let stand in the fridge for 1 hr.

Heat half the olive oil in a saucepan and
brown the onion and garlic.

Add the diced tomato, spices, vinegar, sugar
and the other half of olive oil.
Leave to simmer for 15 min until you
obtain a thick consistency.

Let cool.

Season with salt, pepper and Tabasco sauce.

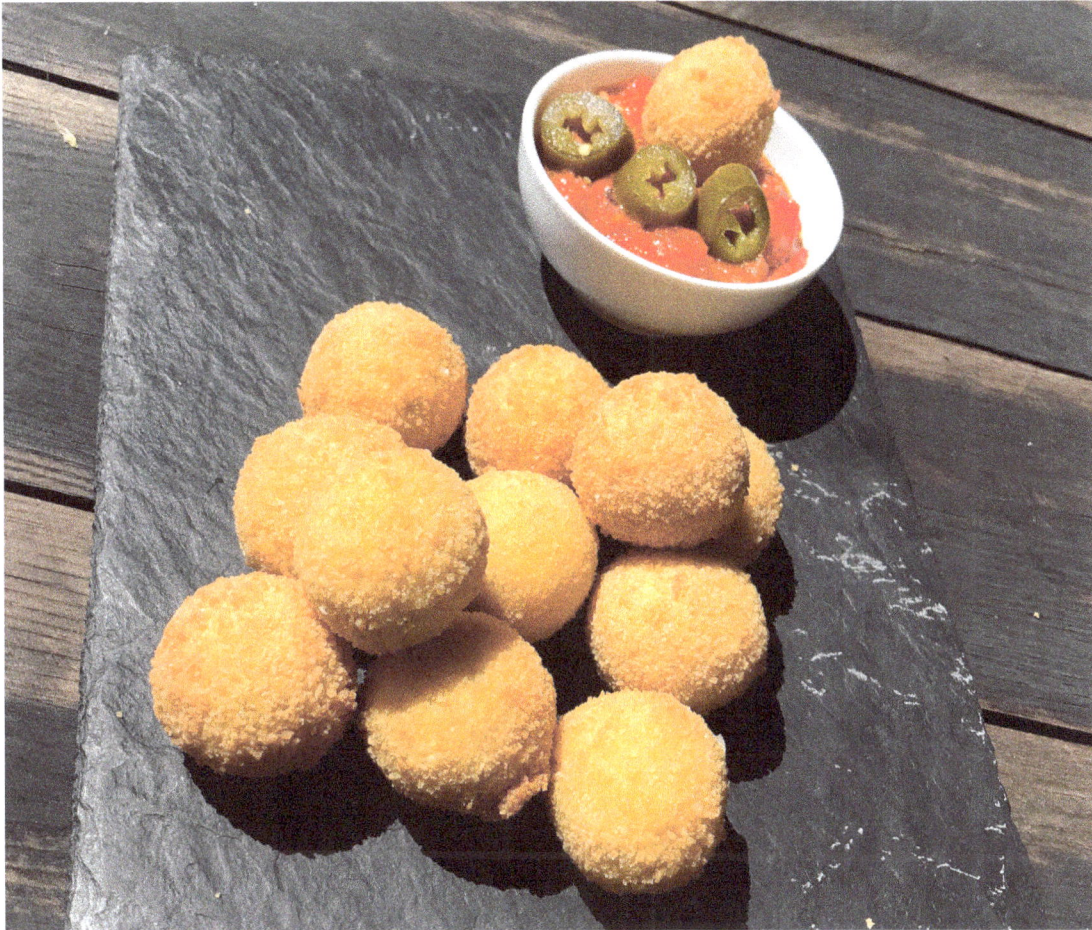

Sprinkle your cheese balls with flour and shake well.

Double-bread the cheese balls (flour-egg-breadcrumbs-egg-breadcrumbs).

Heat a little frying oil to 175°C and fry the cheese balls for about 1 min 30 sec.

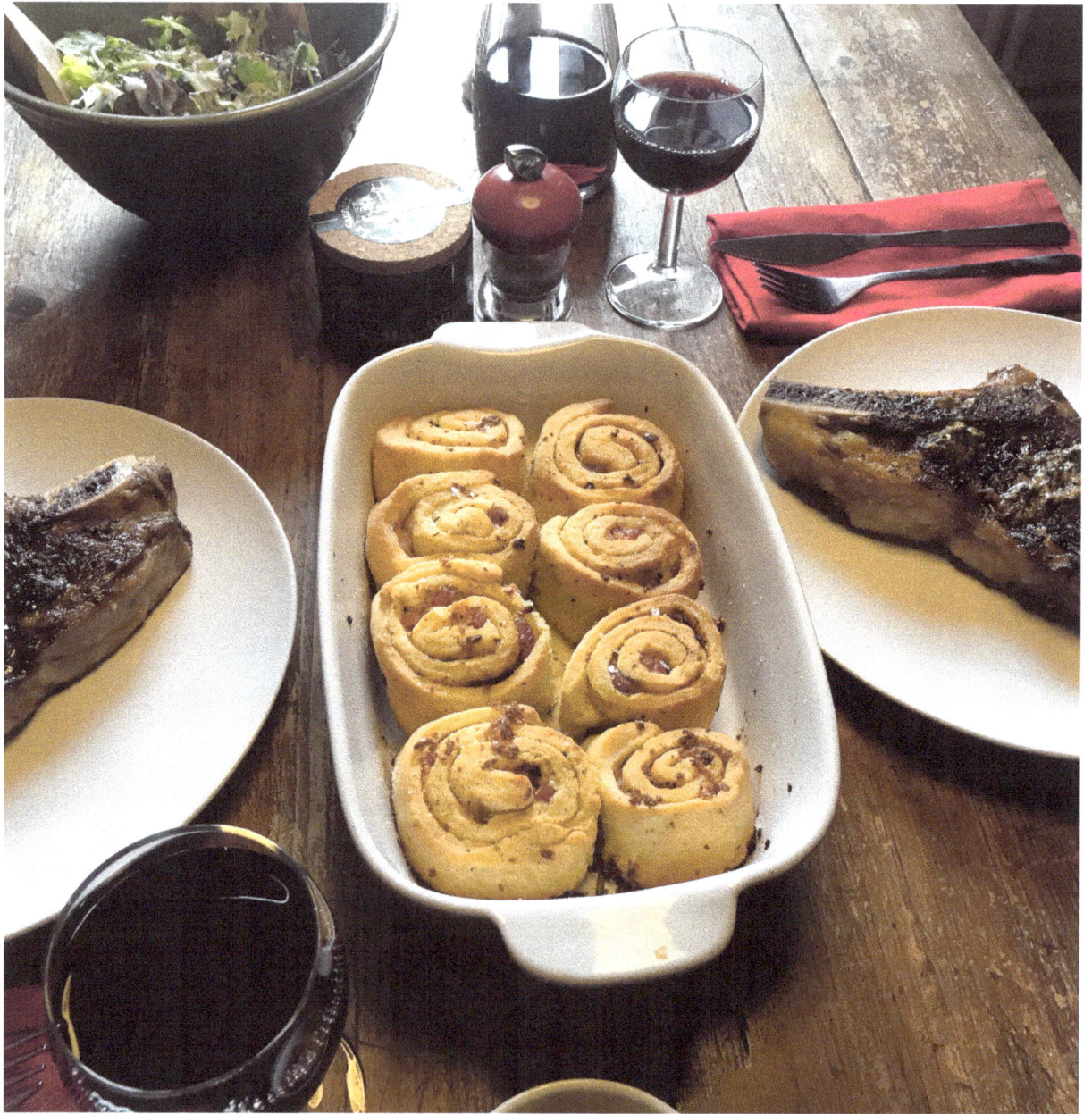

Savory Swiss rolls with bacon and rosemary

260g flour
1/2 cube of yeast (or 1 tsp of dried yeast)
150ml lukewarm milk
40g soft butter
1 tsp salt
1/2 tsp sugar
2 twigs rosemary, chopped
50ml olive oil
2 cloves of garlic, chopped
50g bacon
Piment d'Espelette, French chilli powder

Soak the yeast in the lukewarm milk with the sugar.
Prepare a dough with the flour, soft butter, salt
and milk mixture. Leave to rise for 45 min.

Preheat your oven to 200°C.

Mix the chopped garlic with the olive oil.

Roll out the dough and brush with half the
garlic olive oil. Place the bacon on the dough,
sprinkle with piment d'Espelette and rosemary.

Roll up the dough and cut it into 8 parts.
Brush a baking dish with olive oil and place
the dough rounds on it. Let rise for another 15 min.

Bake for 25 min.

Brush with olive oil.

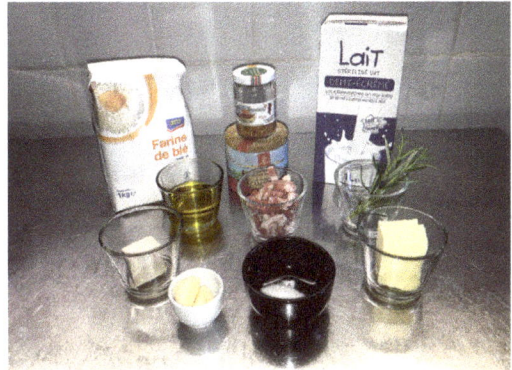

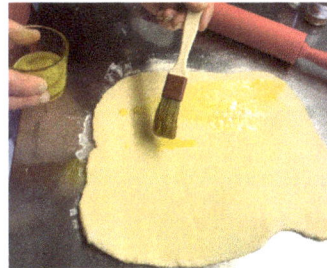

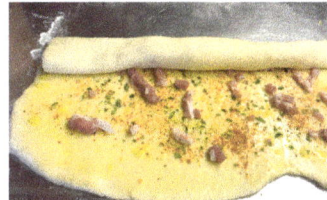

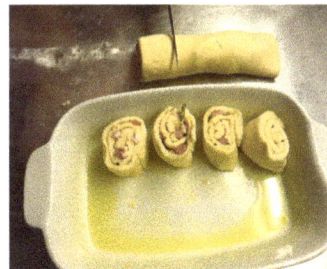

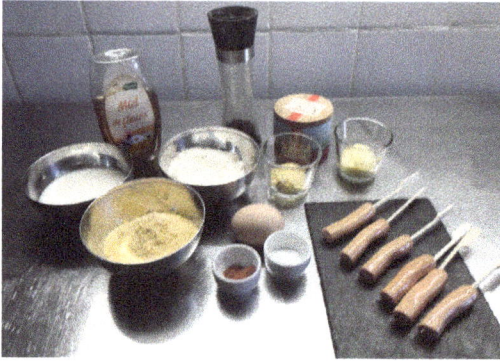

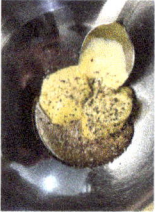

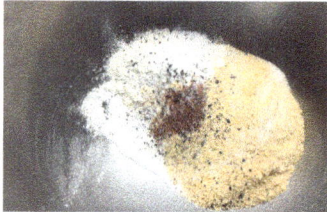

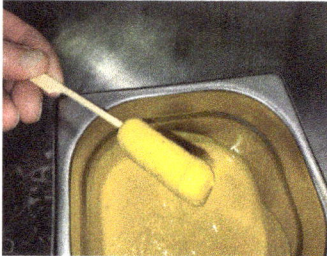

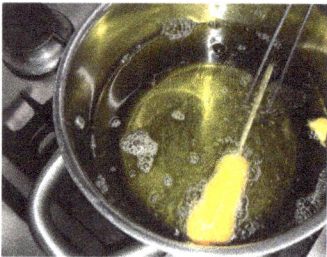

Corn dogs

3 frankfurter sausages
75g flour
75g corn flour
140ml milk
1 egg
1 tbsp honey
1 tsp baking powder
1 tsp chilli powder
Salt, pepper
*
1 tbsp mayonnaise
1 tbsp mustard
Honey

Cut the sausages in half and put them
on wooden skewers.

Prepare a batter with the flour, corn flour,
baking powder, milk, egg, honey and chilli powder.
Season with salt and pepper.

Heat a little frying oil in a saucepan.

Dip the sausages in the batter and fry them
for about 1 min 30 sec.

Mix the mayonnaise and mustard and
season with honey, salt and pepper.

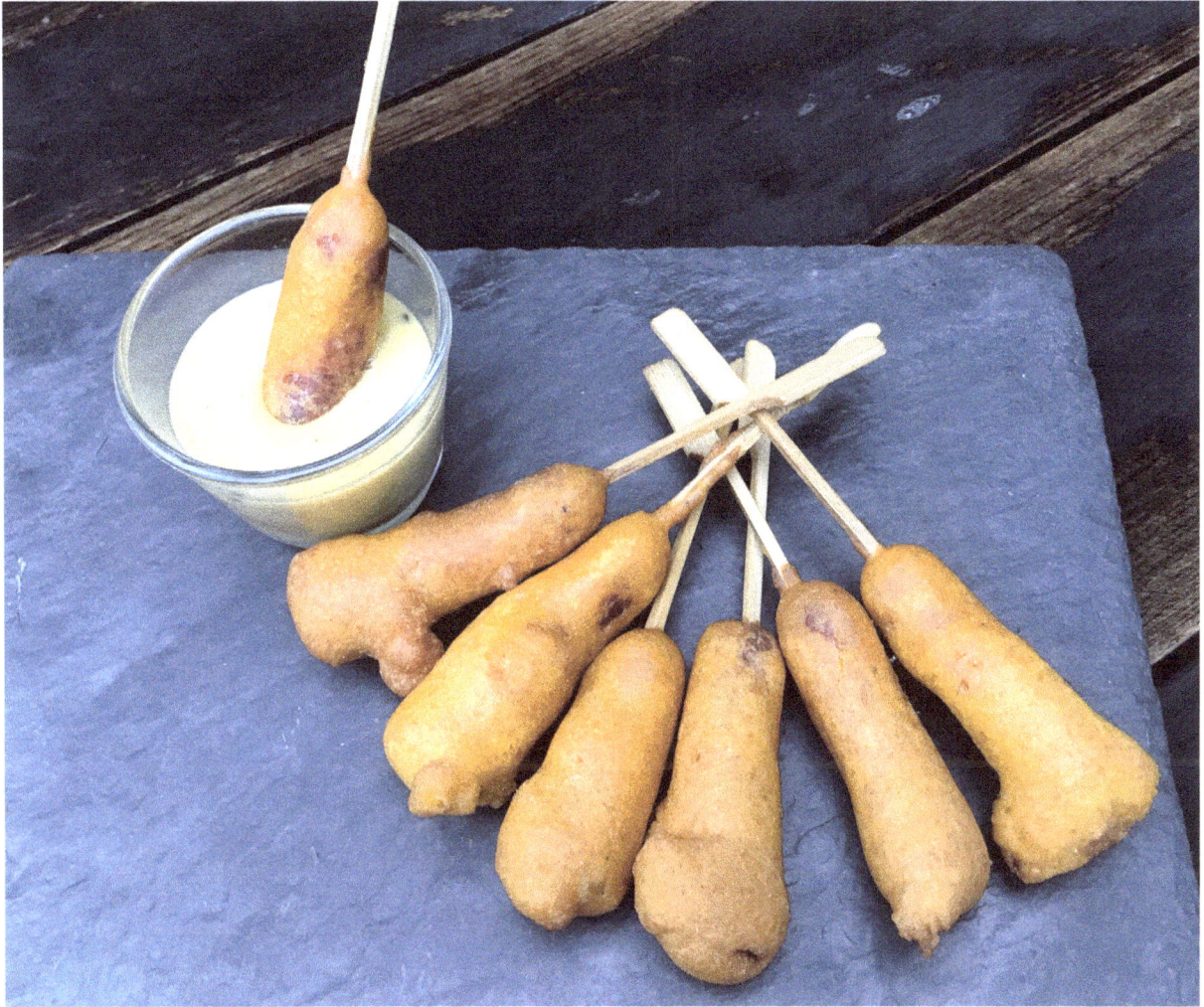

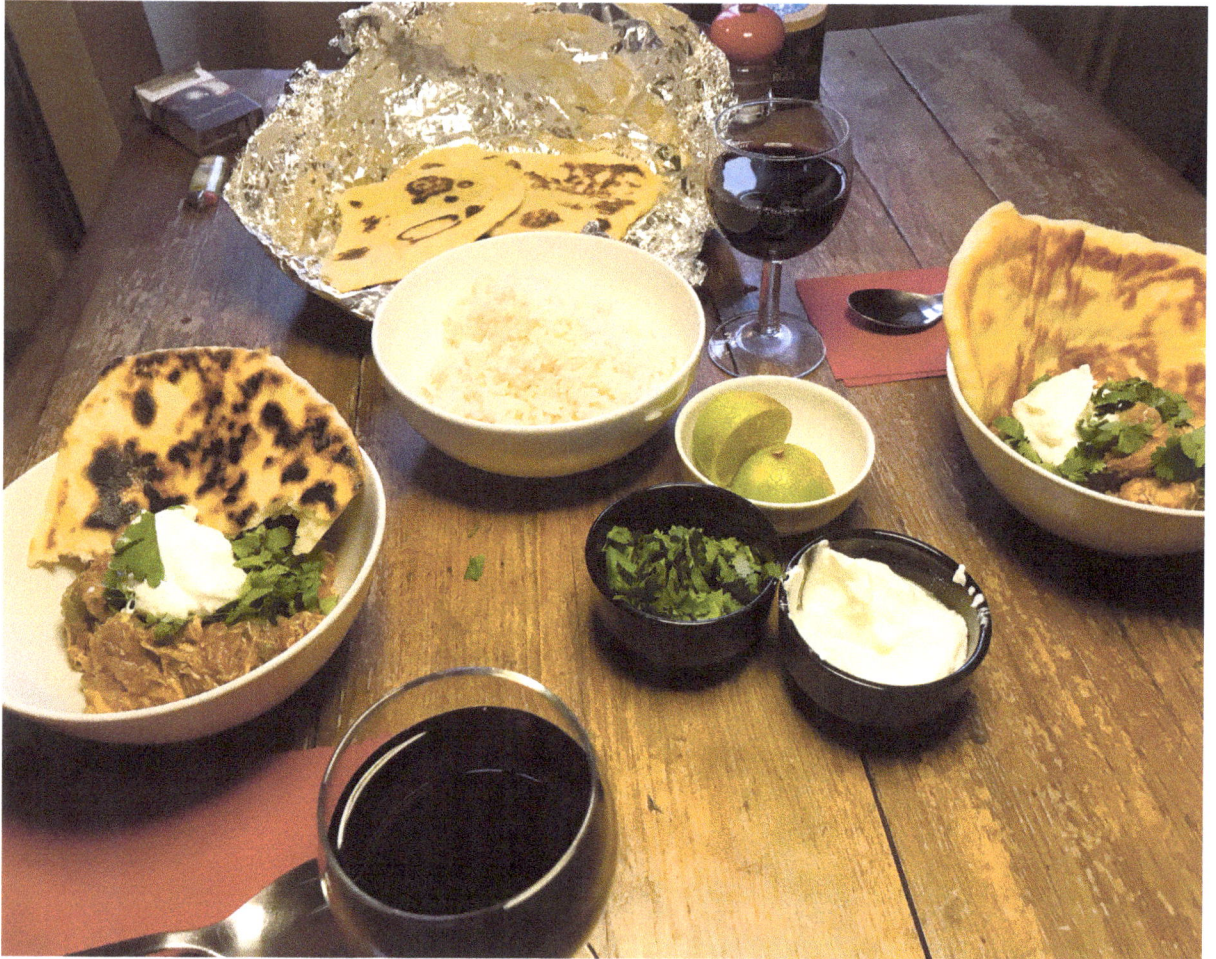

Garlic naan bread

250g flour
1 tsp yeast
1 tsp sugar
75g Greek yogurt
100ml lukewarm water
2 tbsp oil
Salt
2 cloves of garlic, chopped

Dissolve the yeast and sugar in the lukewarm water.

Mix the yogurt with the oil.

Prepare a dough with the flour, yeast mixture,
yoghurt mixed with oil and a little salt.
Leave it to rise for 1 hr.

Divide the dough into 4 parts.
Roll out pieces of about 20cm.
Sprinkle with garlic, fold and roll again.
Leave to rise for 15 min.

Heat a pan and place the naan in it.

When the dough starts to bubble, turn it over
and cook the other side for about 2 min.

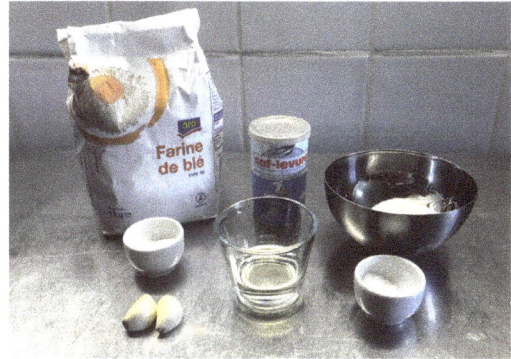

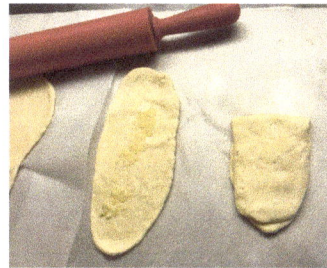

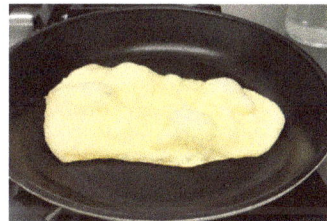

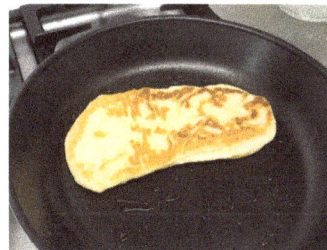

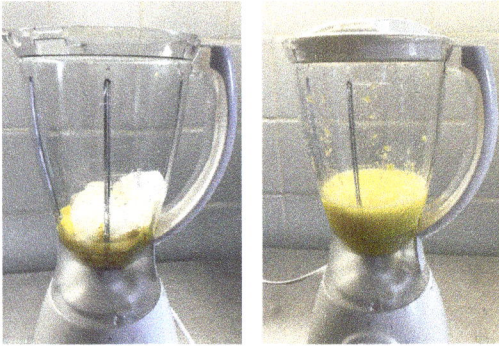

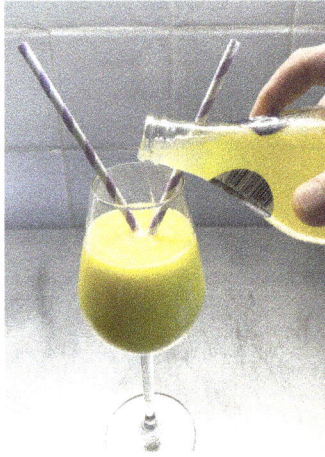

Mangosty

1/2 mango
50ml apple juice
5-7 ice cubes
50ml sparkling water
15ml lime juice
Orangina
Mint

Place the mango, ice cubes, sparkling water,
apple juice and lime juice into a blender.
Mix well until you obtain a smooth liquid.

Pour into a glass.

Top up the glass with Orangina.

Decorate with mint.

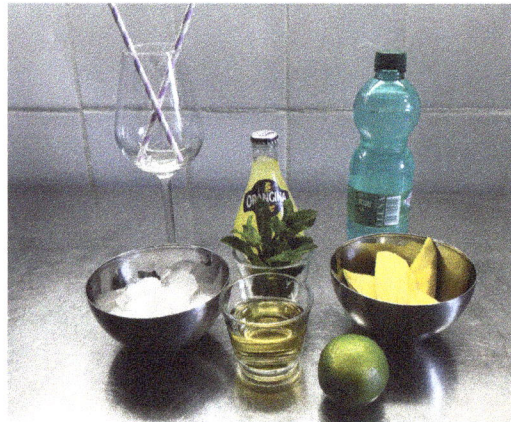

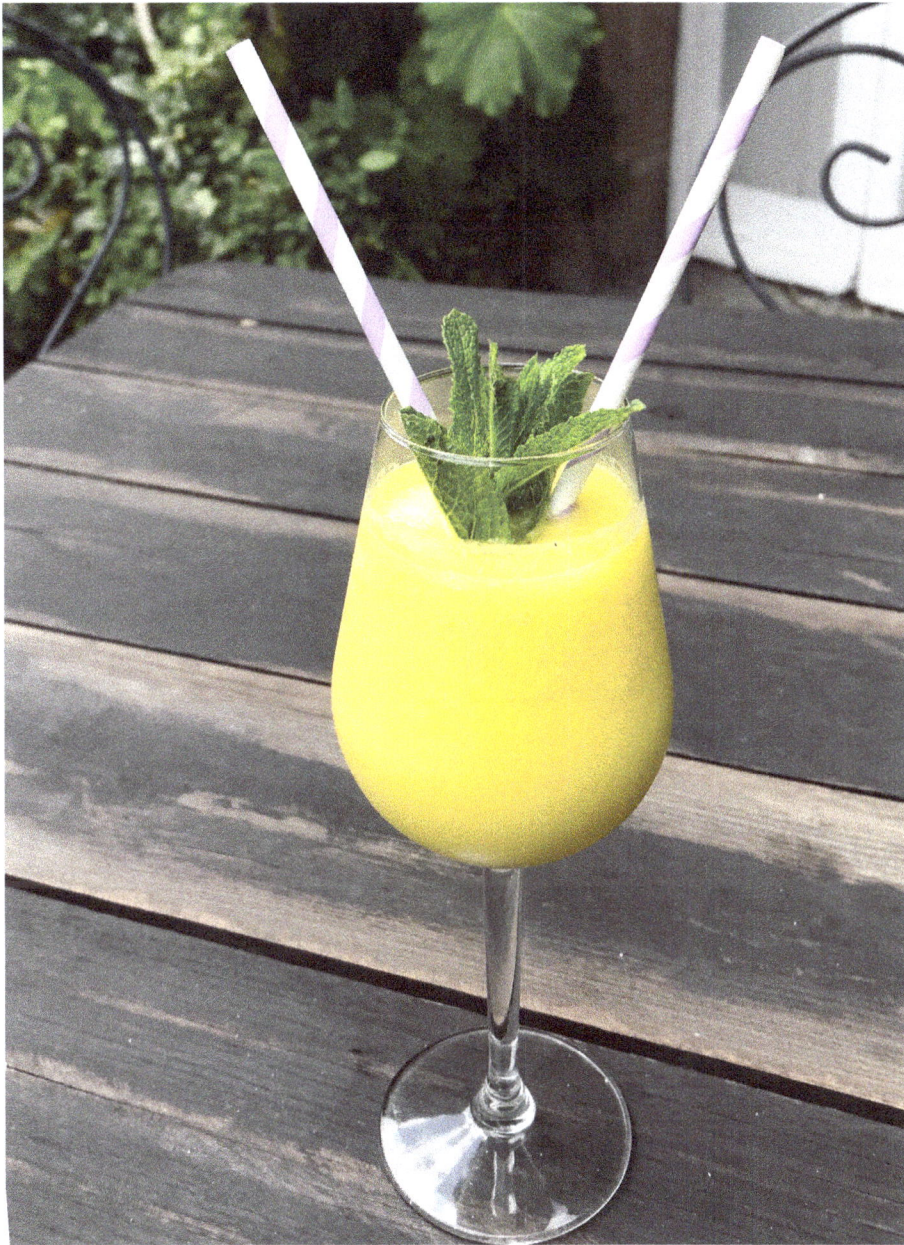

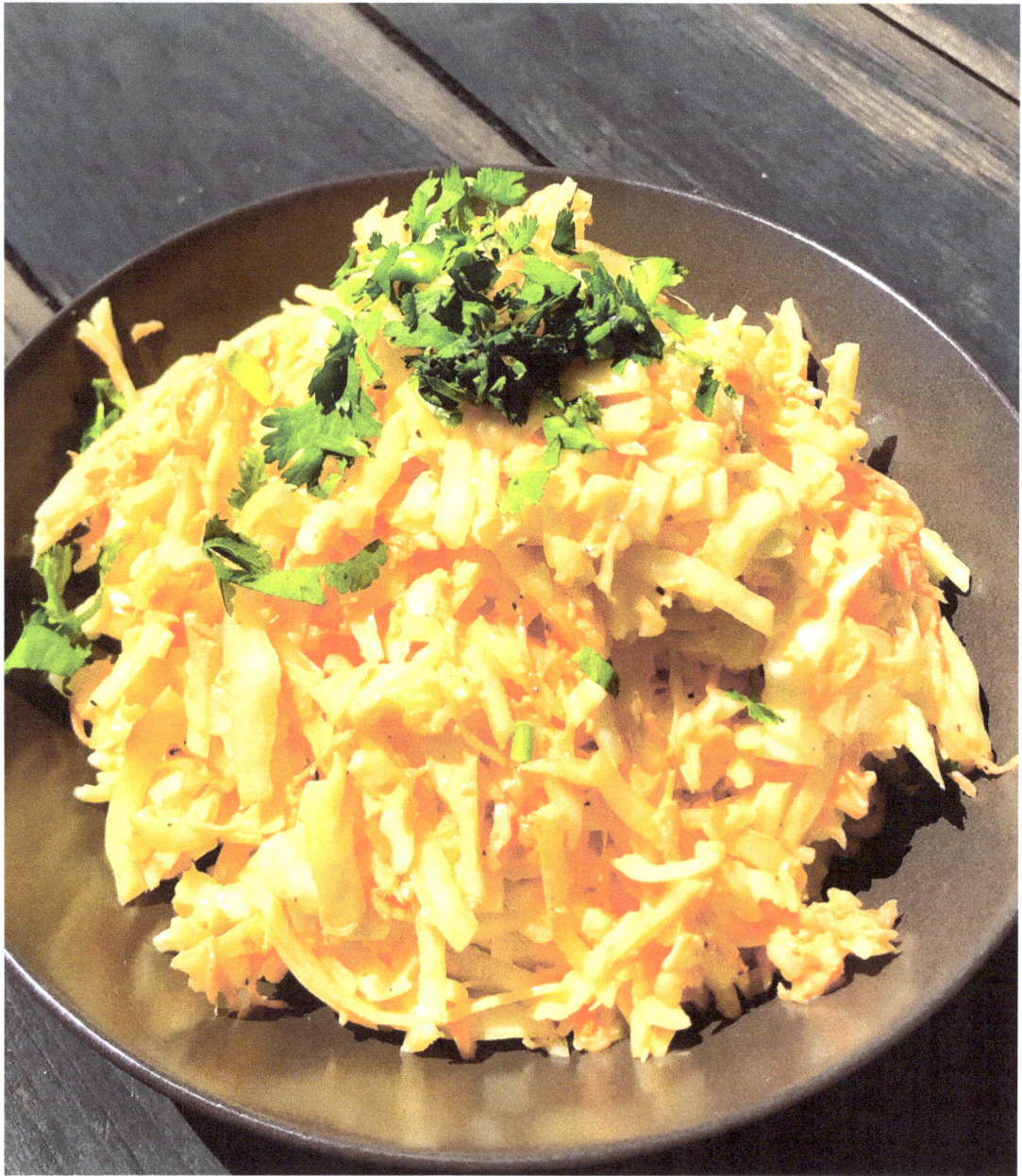

Coleslaw

1/2 white cabbage
3 carrots, grated
1 small onion, diced
Juice of a lime
1 tbsp mayonnaise
1 tbsp crème fraîche
1 tbsp sugar
1/2 tbsp white vinegar
1 tsp mustard
Salt, pepper
Tabasco sauce (optional)

Cut the white cabbage into thin strips.
Add the grated carrots.

Mix together the mayonnaise, crème
fraîche, mustard, vinegar, sugar,
lime juice and onion.

Season with salt and pepper.

Mix the white cabbage well with the sauce.

Leave in the fridge for at least 2 hrs.

Season again with salt, pepper,
sugar and Tabasco.

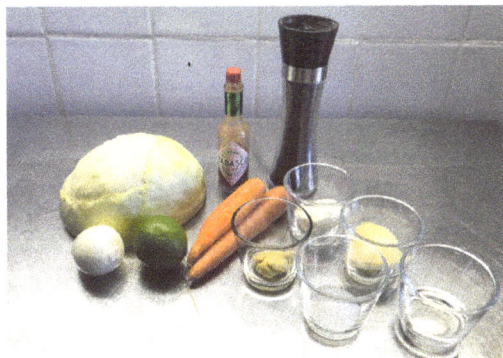

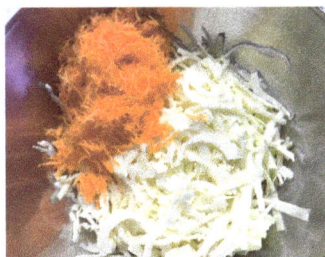

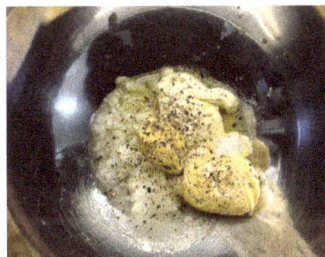

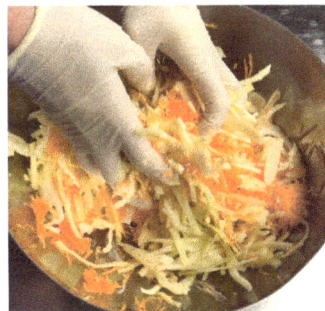

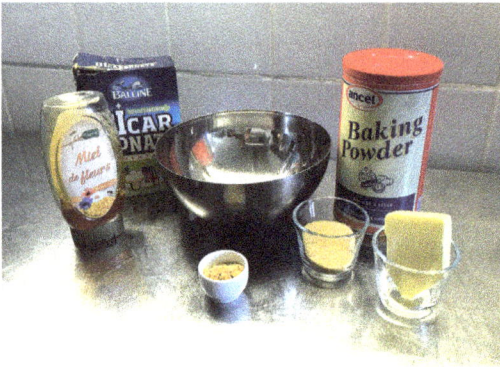

Gingernut cookies

110g flour
50g butter
50g honey
40g cane sugar
1 tsp ground ginger
1 tsp baking soda
1/2 tsp baking powder

Preheat your oven to 180°C.

Mix all the dry ingredients.
Add honey and butter and make a dough.

Roll the dough in cling film and let it
rest in the fridge for about 15 min.

Cut the dough into 16 pieces and flatten
them the help of a spoon or your hand.

Bake the cookies for about 12–15 min
(not 20 mins like we did –
it was a bit too long :)

Leave the cookies to cool.

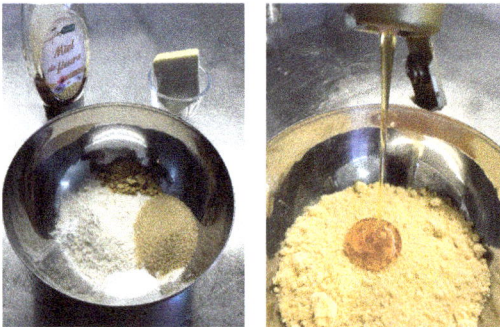

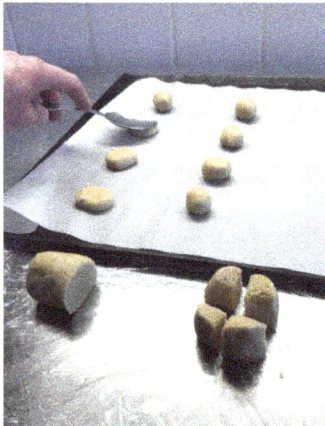

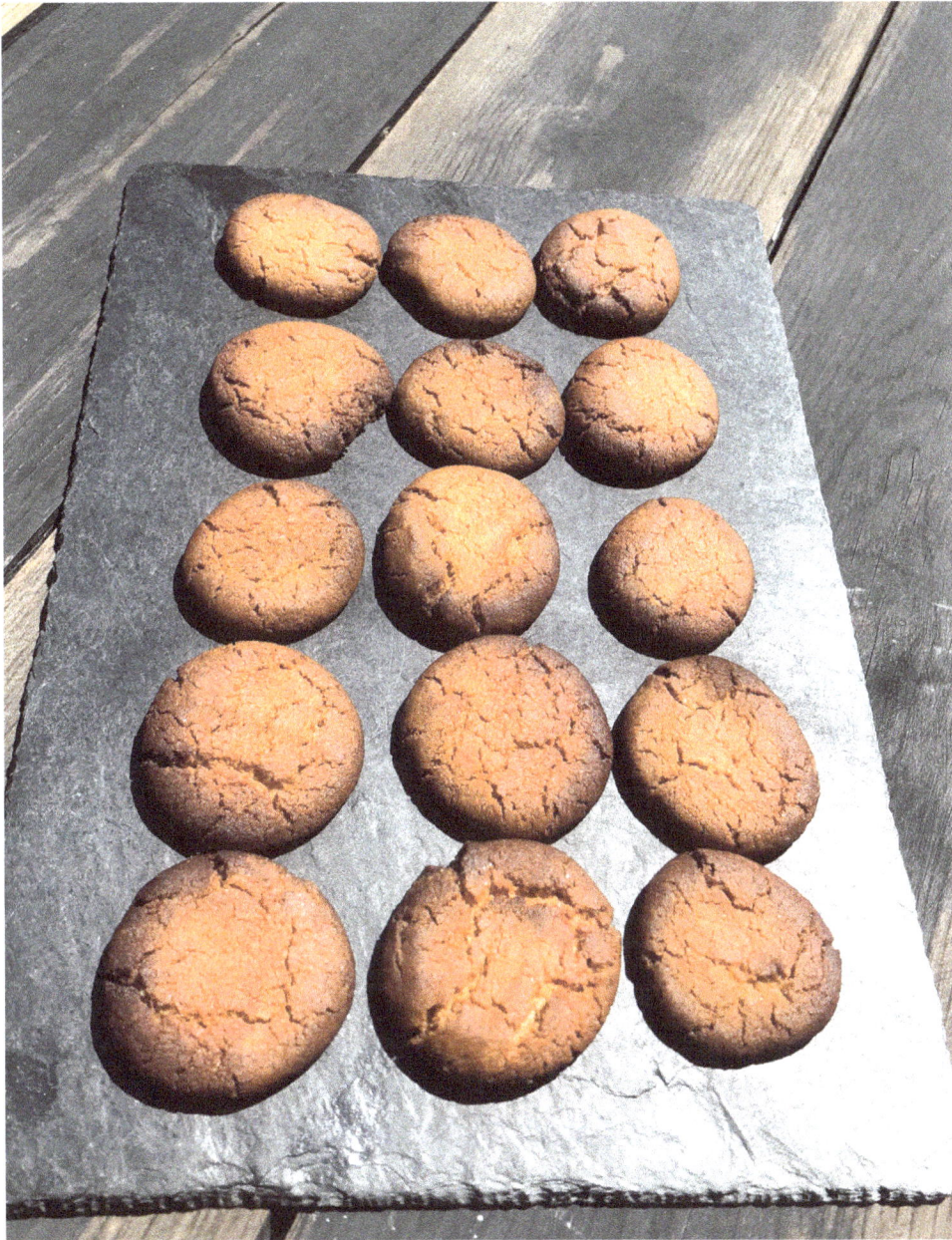

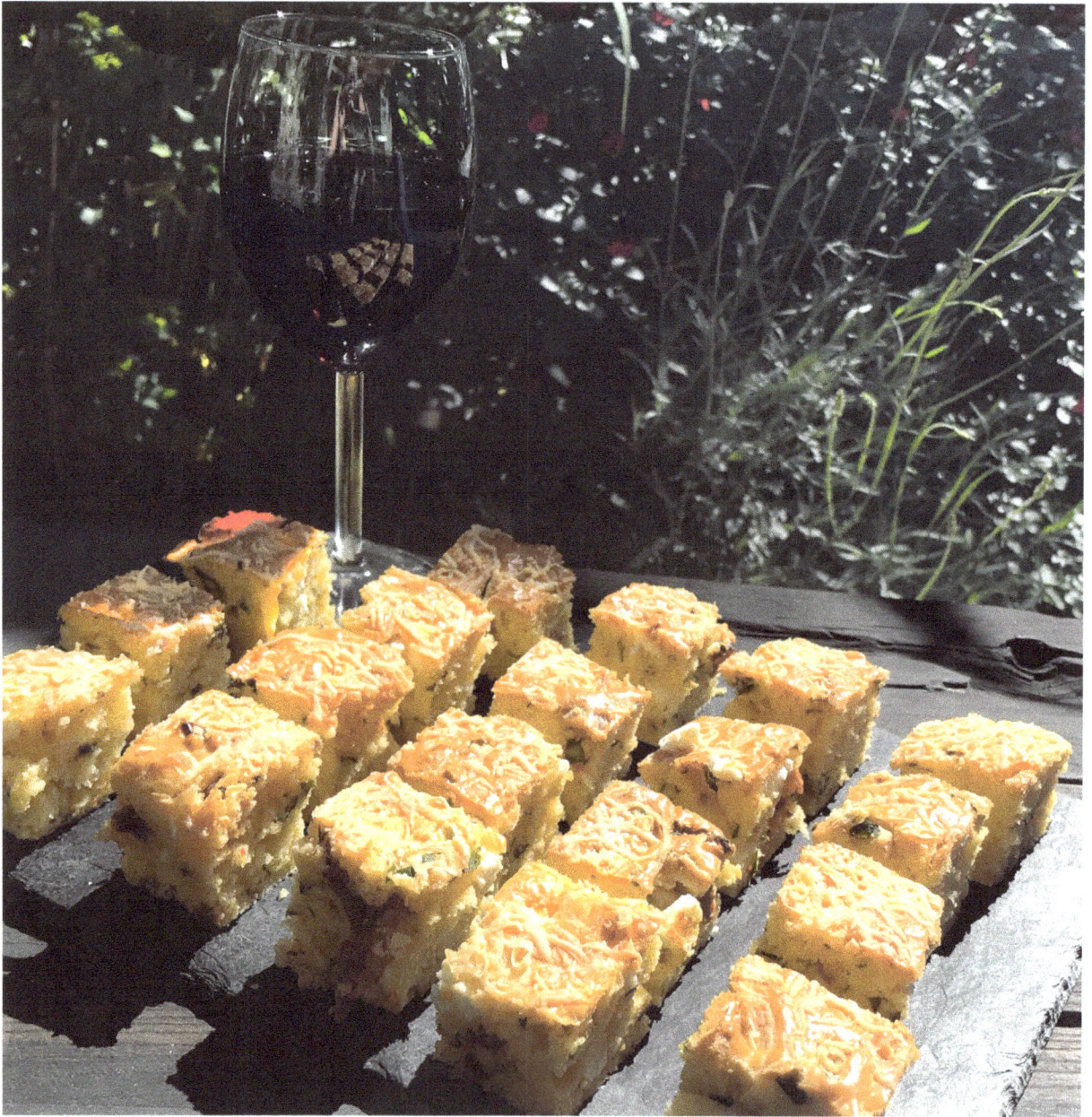

Mini aperitif savory cakes

240g flour
3 eggs
90ml milk
80ml olive oil
40g yogurt
2 tsp baking powder
Piment d'Espelette (optional)
120g feta cheese
50g sundried tomatoes,
20g basil
2 garlic cloves, chopped
20g grated Parmesan cheese

Cut the feta into small cubes and
the basil leaves into thin strips.

Preheat your oven to 175°C.

Prepare a batter with the flour, eggs, olive oil, yogurt,
and baking powder. Add the sundried tomatoes, feta,
garlic and basil. Season with salt, pepper and piment
d'Espelette. Sprinkle with the Parmesan.

Pour into a small, deep baking tray lined with
baking paper. In a slightly larger baking tray, pour
400ml of water and place the smaller baking tray in it.
(If you don't have two baking sheets, you can also put a
bowl of water in your oven.)

Bake for 35 min.

Let it cool before cutting into small pieces.

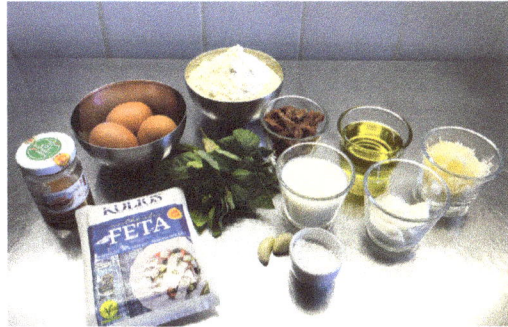

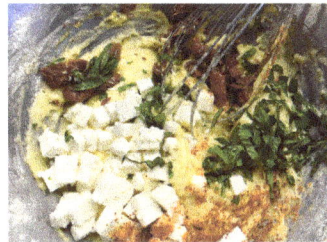

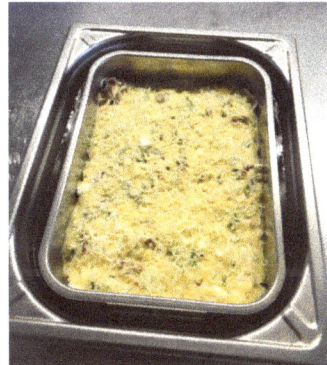

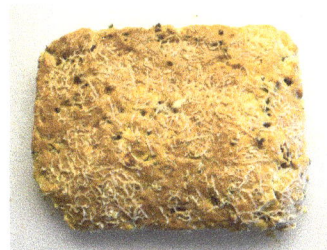

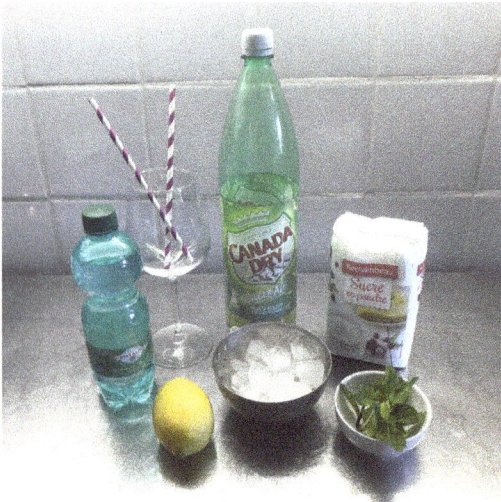

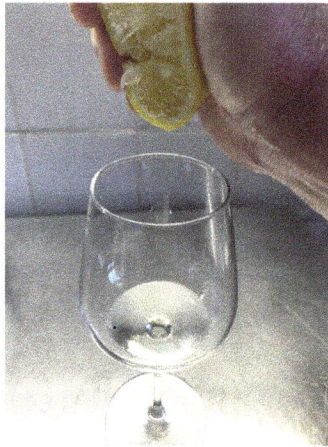

Piégut mule

150ml ginger ale or Canada Dry
50ml sparkling water
100ml water
100g sugar
3–4 mint leaves
1 lemon
Ice cubes

Heat the water and sugar in a saucepan
and reduce to the consistency of syrup.

Let cool.

Pour 8cl of the syrup into a glass.
(You can keep the rest in the fridge
for other recipes.)

Add the lemon juice and mint.

Fill the glass with sparkling water
and ginger ale.

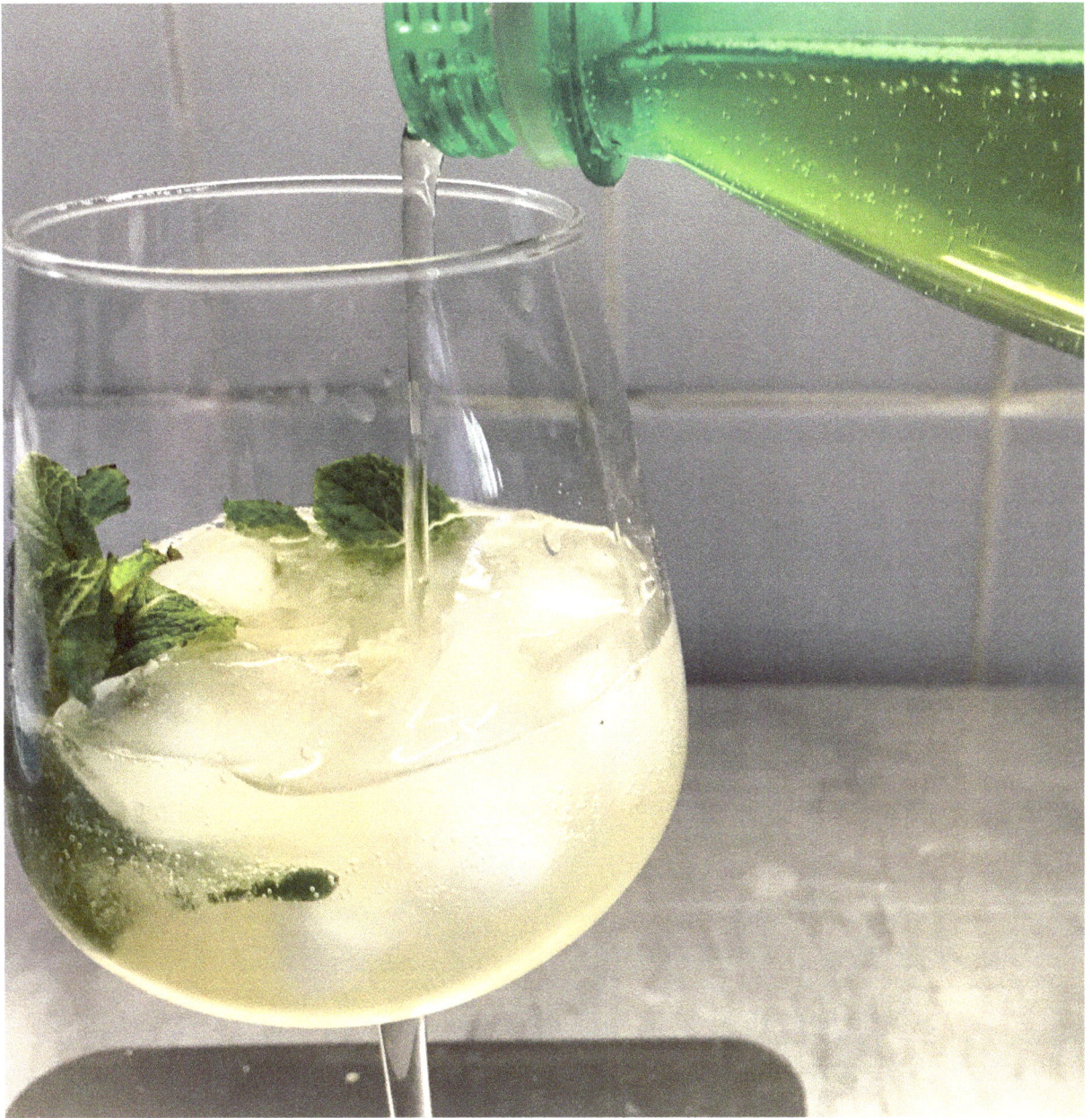

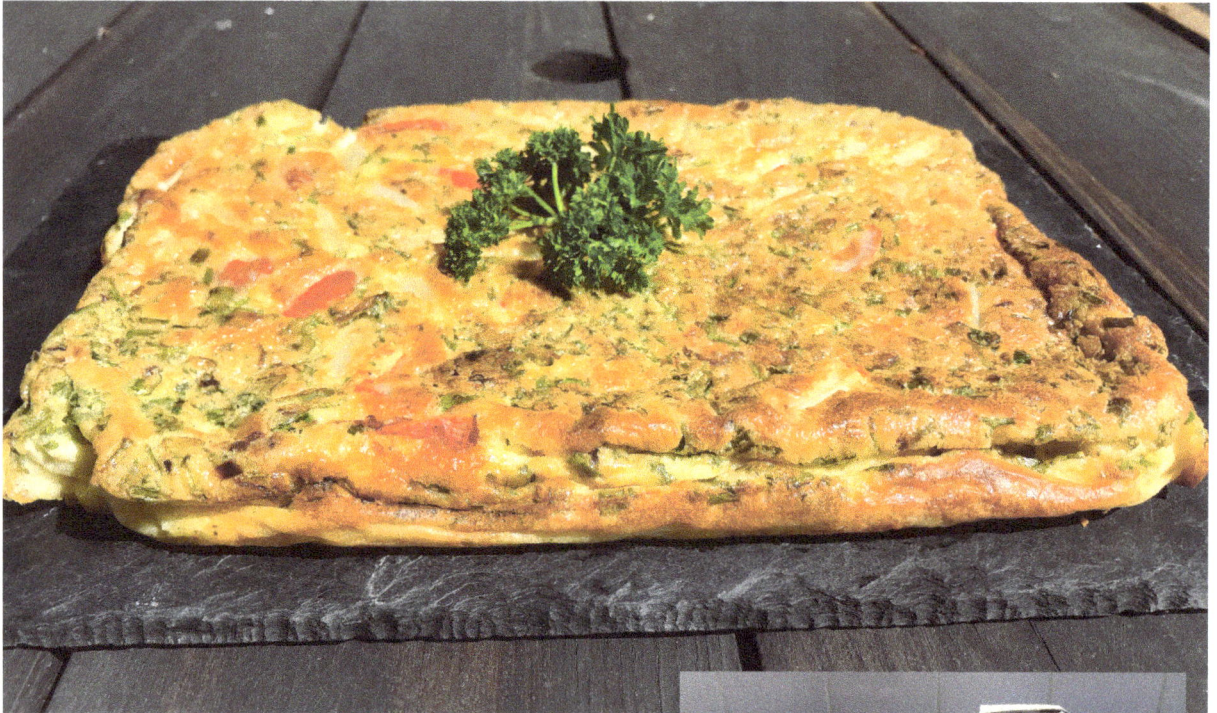

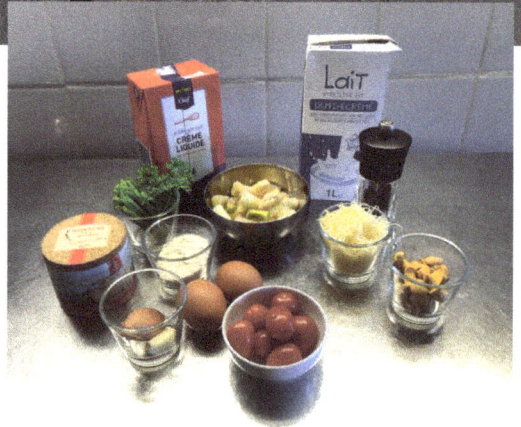

Asparagus and chanterelle clafoutis

150g asparagus, cut into small pieces
80–100g chanterelle mushrooms
1 clove of garlic, chopped
1 shallot, diced
5 cherry tomatoes, cut in half
3 eggs
125ml milk
250ml cream
30g grated Parmesan cheese
30g flour
Parsley, chives

Blanch the asparagus pieces in boiling water.

Preheat your oven to 175°C.

Brown the onions and garlic in a pan
with a little oil. Add the chanterelles and
fry them for 2–3 min.

Mix the milk, cream, eggs, Parmesan,
flour and herbs.

Add the asparagus, chanterelles and tomatoes.

Season with salt and pepper.

Pour into a deep lined baking tray.

Cook for 15–20 min.

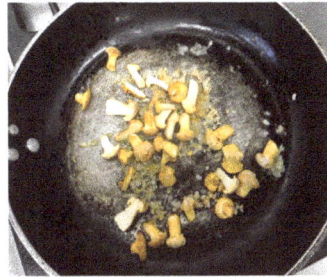

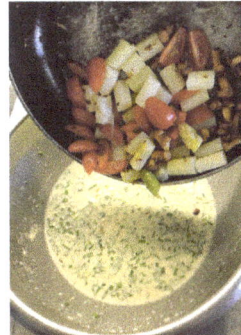

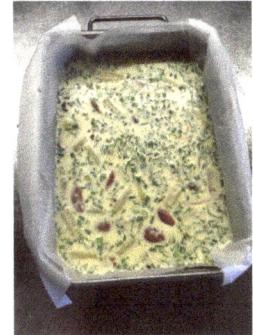

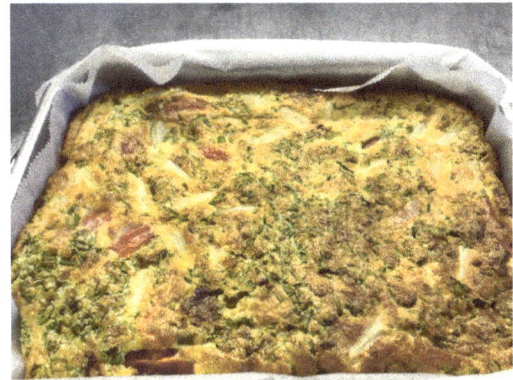

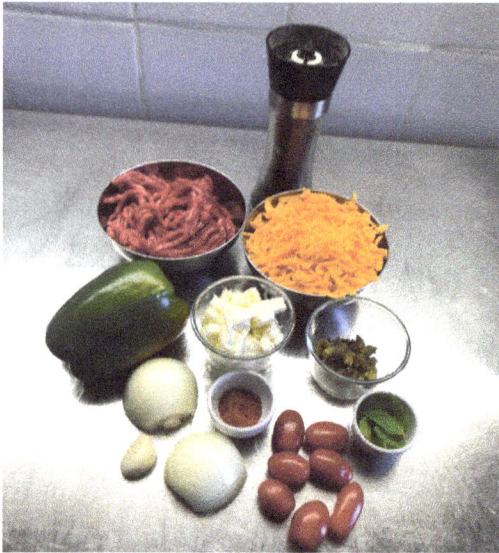

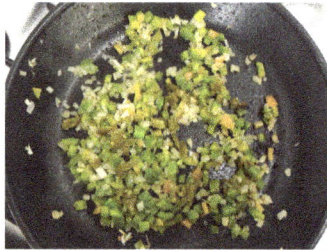

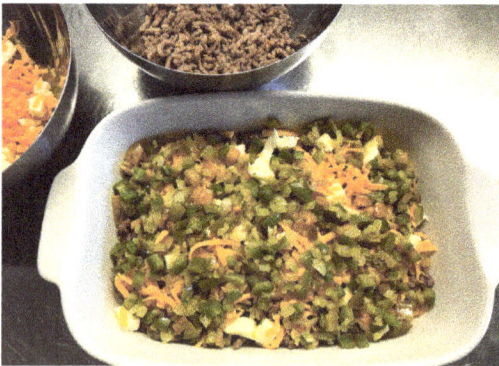

Queso fundido

200g minced meat
150g grated cheddar cheese
75g mozzarella cheese, diced
1 green pepper, diced
1 diced onion
1 clove of garlic, minced
3–5 slices chopped jalapeño (or more)
5–6 oregano leaves
1/2 tsp hot pepper
Salt, pepper

Preheat your oven to 220°C.

In a frying pan, cook the minced meat.
Season with salt, pepper, hot pepper and
oregano, and set aside.

In the same pan, brown the diced peppers, onion and
garlic for about 4 min. Add the chopped jalapenos.

Mix the two cheeses. Sprinkle 1/4 of the cheese
in a baking pan. Cover with 2/3 of the minced meat.
Sprinkle with 1/4 of the cheese. Add the vegetables and
another 1/4 of the cheese. Cover with the rest of the
minced meat and finish with the last 1/4 of cheese.

Bake for about 10 min, until cheese is bubbly.

Garnish with small tomatoes, coriander,
and slices of jalapenos.

Serve with nachos.

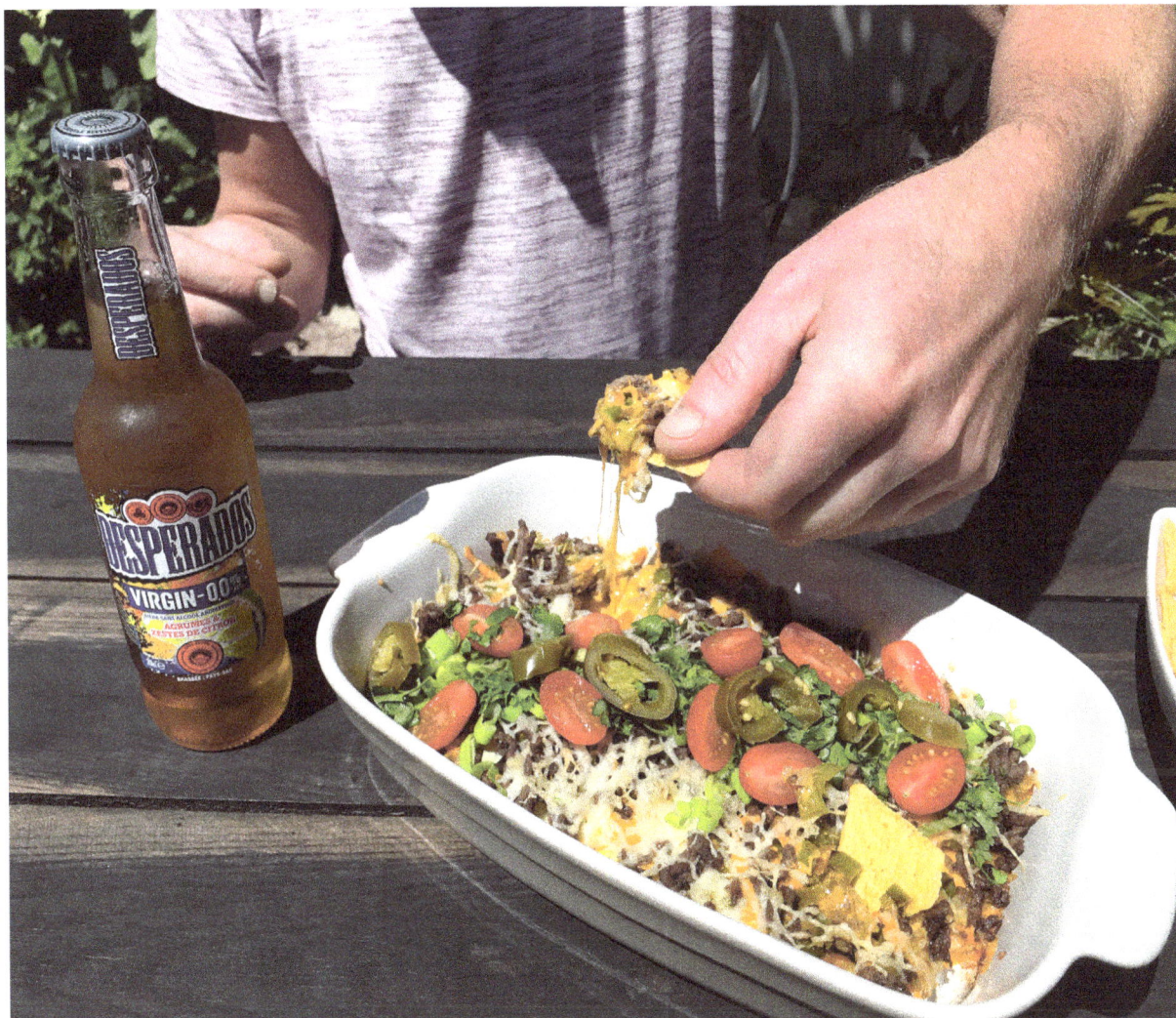

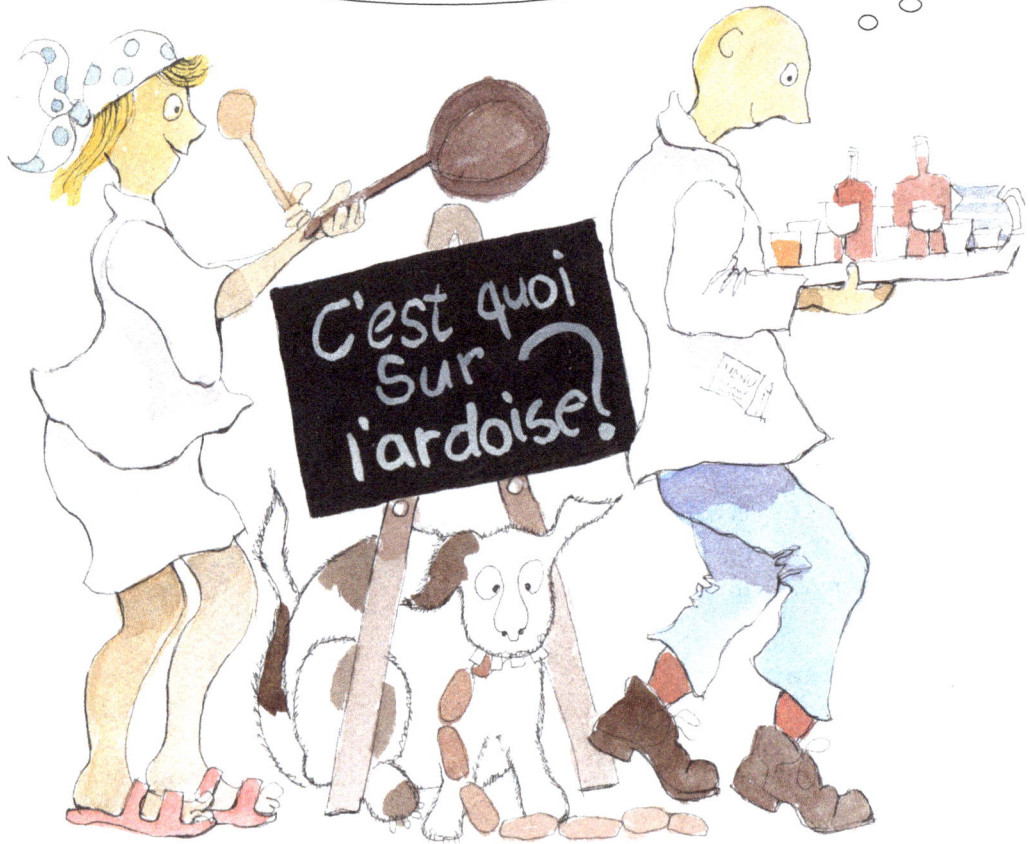

Thank you!

First of all, we would like to thank our loyal customers
whose support enabled us to keep our restaurant open,
despite restrictions, throughout the lockdown. Thanks also
to Chuck and Lynne Grieve, our publishers, who
encouraged us to turn the recipes on our Facebook
page into this little book.

For the illustrations, we are grateful for the
creativity of Howard, and Hugo Woods.

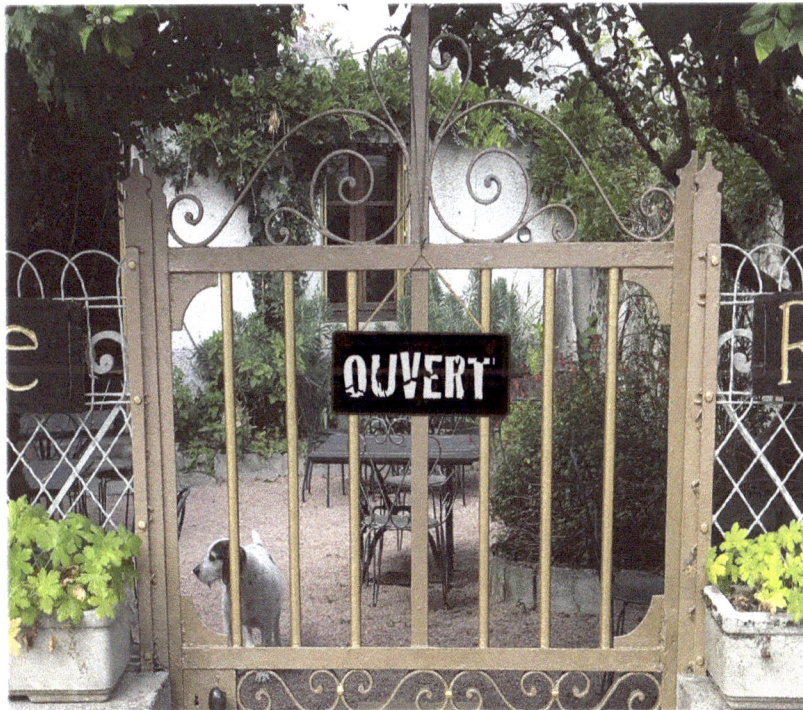

Notes

www.ingramcontent.com/pod-product-compliance
Lightning Source LLC
Chambersburg PA
CBHW050257090426
42734CB00022B/3480